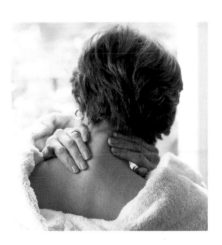

AROMATHERAPY
A STEP-BY-STEP GUIDE FOR WOMEN

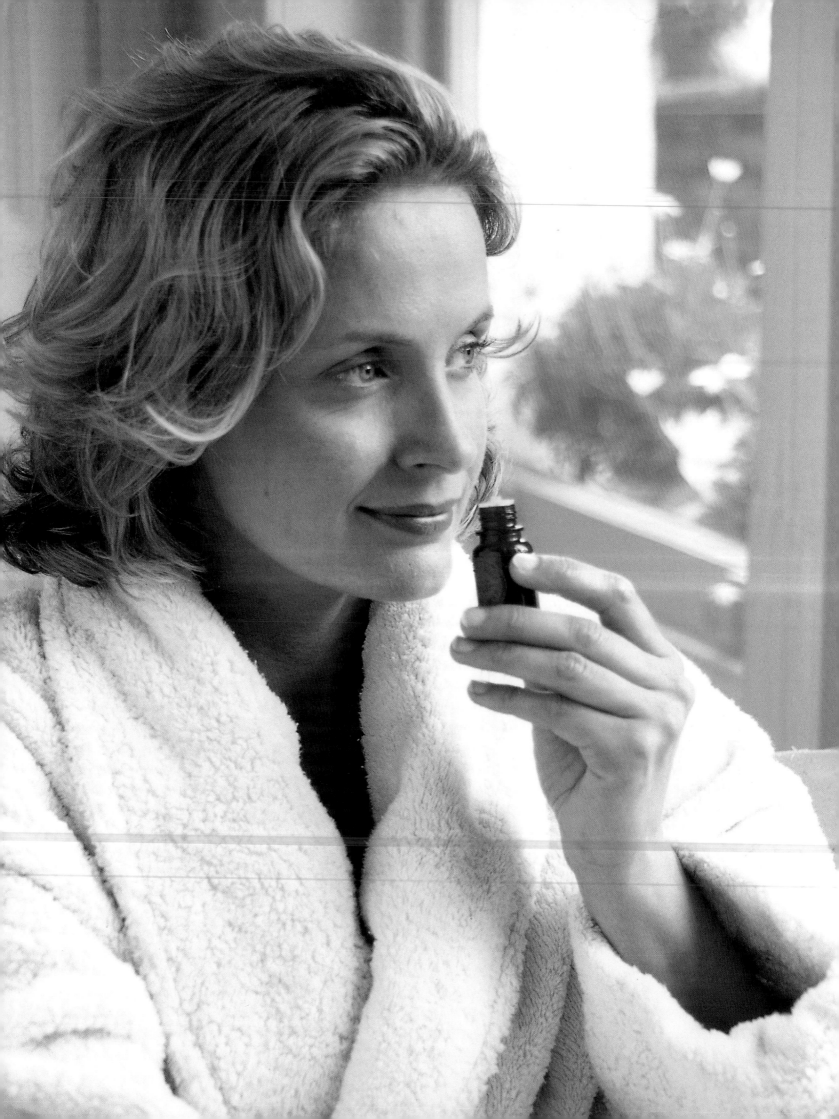

AROMATHERAPY
A STEP-BY-STEP GUIDE FOR WOMEN

HOW TO USE ESSENTIAL OILS FOR IMPROVED HEALTH AND VITALITY
THROUGH ALL STAGES OF LIFE, WITH 200 PRACTICAL PHOTOGRAPHS

SHIRLEY PRICE

HERMES
HOUSE

This edition is published by Hermes House, an imprint of Anness Publishing Ltd, Hermes House, 88–89 Blackfriars Road, London SE1 8HA; tel. 020 7401 2077; fax 020 7633 9499

www.hermeshouse.com; www.annesspublishing.com

If you like the images in this book and would like to investigate using them for publishing, promotions or advertising, please visit our website www.practicalpictures.com for more information.

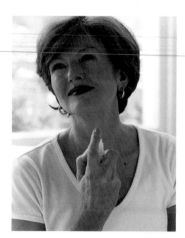

Publisher **Joanna Lorenz**
Managing Editor **Judith Simons**
Project Editor **Sarah Ainley**
Copy Editor **Raje Airey**
Designer **Lisa Tai**
Photographer **Michelle Garrett**
Photographer's Assistant **Charlotte Christie**
Indexer **Helen Snaith**
Editorial Reader **Hayley Kerr**
Production Controller **Don Campaniello**

Additional photography
t = top; b = bottom; c = centre; l = left; r = right
Harry Smith Collection pp14tc, 15tl;
Len Price pp21tl, 22cb; **Life File** pp69r, 88tr.

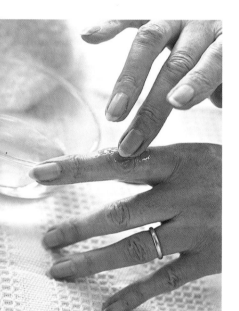

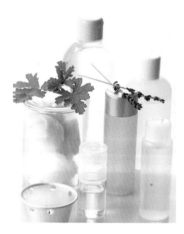

Previously published as *Aromatherapy for Women*

Ethical Trading Policy

Because of our ongoing ecological investment programme, you, as our customer, can have the pleasure and reassurance of knowing that a tree is being cultivated on your behalf to naturally replace the materials used to make the book you are holding. For further information about this scheme, go to www.annesspublishing.com/trees

Note to reader/disclaimer

Although the advice and information in this book are believed to be accurate and true at the time of going to press, neither the authors nor the publisher can accept any legal responsibility or liability for any errors or omissions that may have been made nor for any inaccuracies nor for any loss, harm or injury that comes about from following instructions or advice in this book.

This book is not intended to replace advice from a qualified medical practitioner. Physical illness, nutritional difficulties and environmental stresses can all cause emotional imbalances which may not respond to appropriate aromatherapy treatment. Essential oils are for minor and chronic problems only. The techniques and suggestions in this book are not intended as a substitute for serious medical or psychotic conditions. Please seek a medical opinion if you have any doubts about your health. Neither the author nor the publisher can accept any liability for failure to follow this advice.

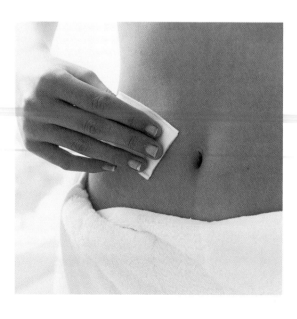

Contents

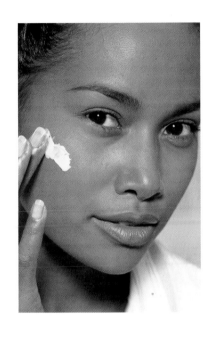

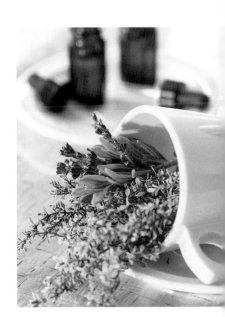

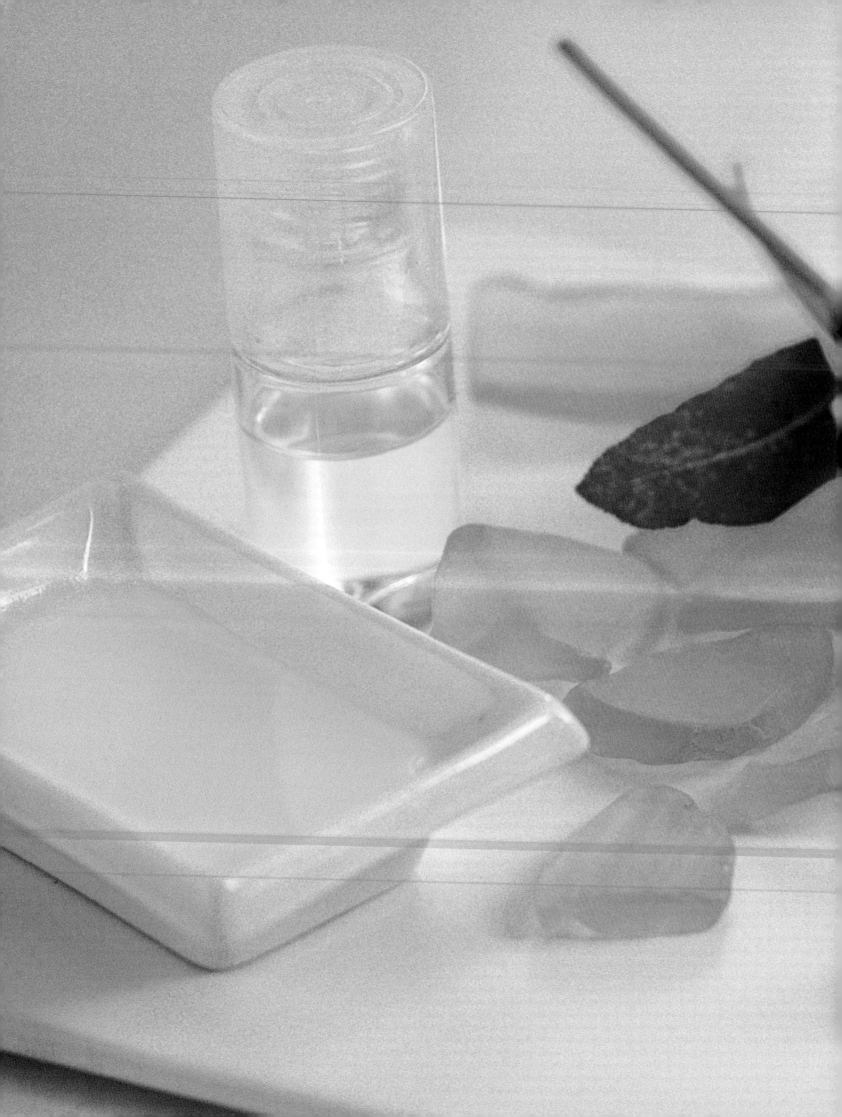

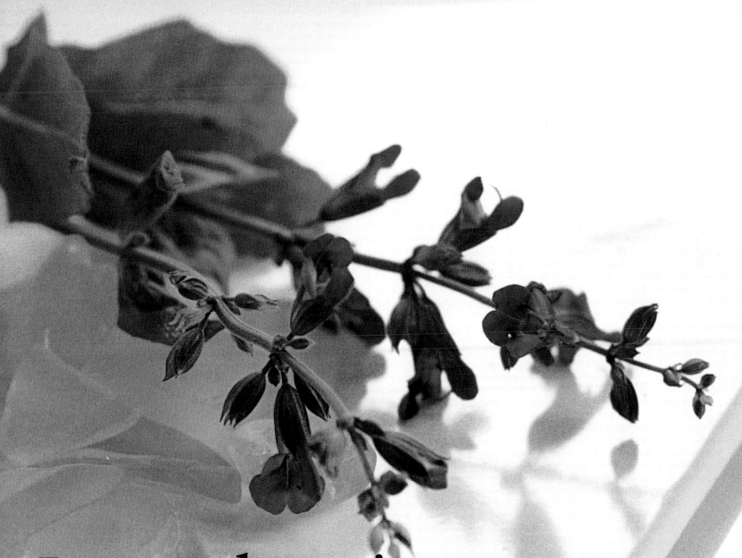

Introduction

He who rules scent rules the heart of man.

From Perfume, Patrick Suskind, 1986.

What is aromatherapy?

Many books have been written on the subject of aromatherapy. This one aims to be a little different in that it will illustrate how any woman can benefit from using essential oils throughout the stages of her life – beginning with the onset of puberty, through pregnancy and her reproductive years, on to the menopause and beyond. The book gives profiles of some of the most commonly used oils and describes how they can be used to treat physical and emotional conditions and to alleviate stress. It gives an overview of essential oils and offers advice for the best methods of use in the home. It also describes how oils can be incorporated into a woman's daily skin and beauty regime. First though, it is important to understand what is meant by aromatherapy, as well as something of how it works.

A popular conception of aromatherapy is as a "massage using essential oils". Although there is a connection between massage and aromatherapy, it is not strictly correct to define one in terms of the other.

Aromatherapy has been defined as "the controlled and knowledgeable use of essential oils for therapeutic purposes". These oils are powerful substances and they should always be handled with care, with professional advice taken where necessary. The essential oils used in aromatherapy are not the same as those used by the perfume and food industries, which standardize or adulterate them for commercial interest. Essential oils for aromatherapy should be natural, with nothing added or taken away.

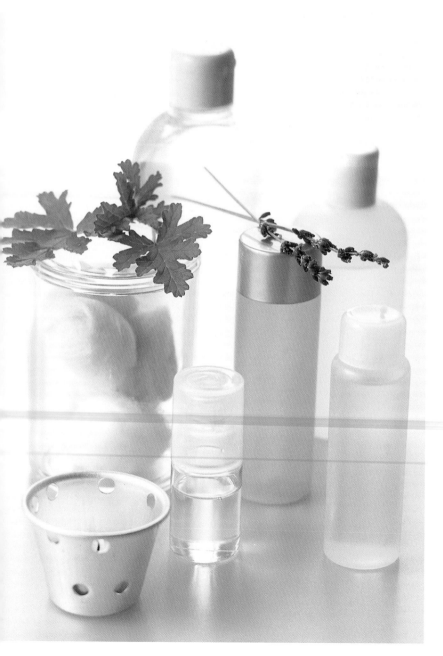

◁ **Many different plant extracts are used in beauty products. An extract is chosen not only for its fragrance, but also for its healing properties.**

▷ **Essential oils can be applied on a compress. Cut up pieces of cotton material and soak them in an oil and water preparation.**

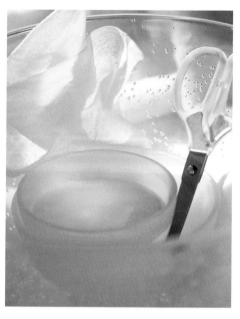

▷ **Vaporizing special aromatherapy candles is an easy way to set the mood for any occasion.**

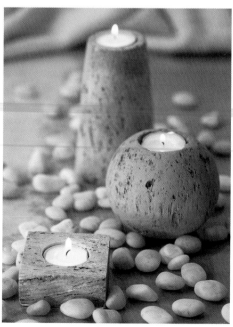
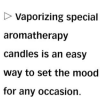

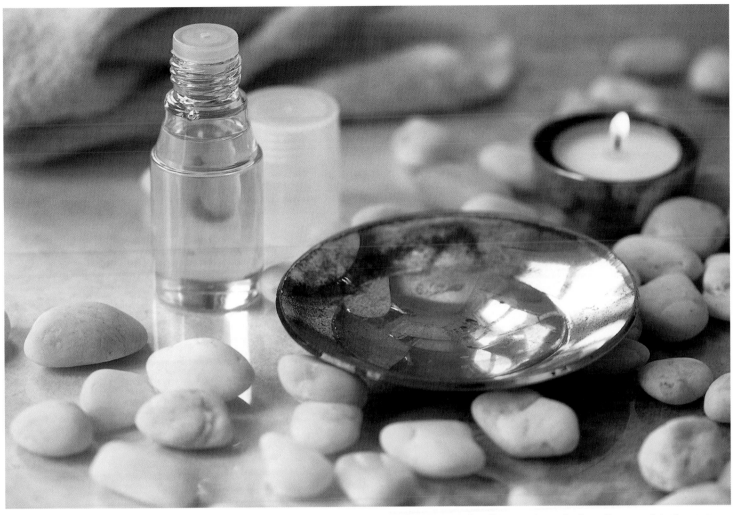

△ Adding a few drops of essential oil to a saucer of water and heating it over a candle flame causes the oil to vaporize and release its aroma into the room.

How to use this book

When essential oils are used for pleasure alone, the choice of oil is usually based on an individual's preferred aroma, and the properties and effects of the oil are not a priority. However, when used to maintain or improve health, the properties and effects are an important part of the choice.

Each essential oil has many properties, and these can affect both body and mind in more than one way. For example, rosemary essential oil has analgesic properties which will benefit headaches, painful digestion and muscular pain. However, rosemary is also a neurotonic, and can relieve general fatigue and stimulate the memory.

At the end of each section of this book is a list of essential oils recommended to help problems associated with that stage in life. Next to each one, from the oil's many assets, are shown the properties relevant to

the particular problem. As an example, where geranium is suggested for athlete's foot, its antifungal quality is listed because this is the property required. In another case, where geranium is suggested for diarrhoea, its anti-inflammatory, antispasmodic and astringent properties are given because these are the relevant properties.

An enhanced result can often be obtained by selecting and using more than one essential oil (two, three or even four different essential oils can be used to make up the required number of drops). The synergy of the blended oils will result in an increase of energy within the mix, when compared to the energy available from one single essential oil.

Having selected the oils you want to use, the chapter on Aromatherapy Techniques will show you how to prepare them for use.

The application techniques suitable for use at home are shown here – application to the skin in a carrier oil, which takes the oils into the bloodstream and all around the body, or by inhalation alone. When we breathe in, some essential oil molecules travel to the lungs to be absorbed into the blood. Other molecules go directly to the brain. This is the quickest route and the most effective way to heal weak or fragile emotions and states of mind, such as stress and depression. The nose not only warms and cleans the inhaled air, but it also enables us to identify substances by their smell. Tiny hairs in the human nose, called cilia, send information via receptor cells to the brain to identify the inhaled molecules. The brain then releases neurochemicals, and these have either a sedative or a tonic effect, depending on the aroma.

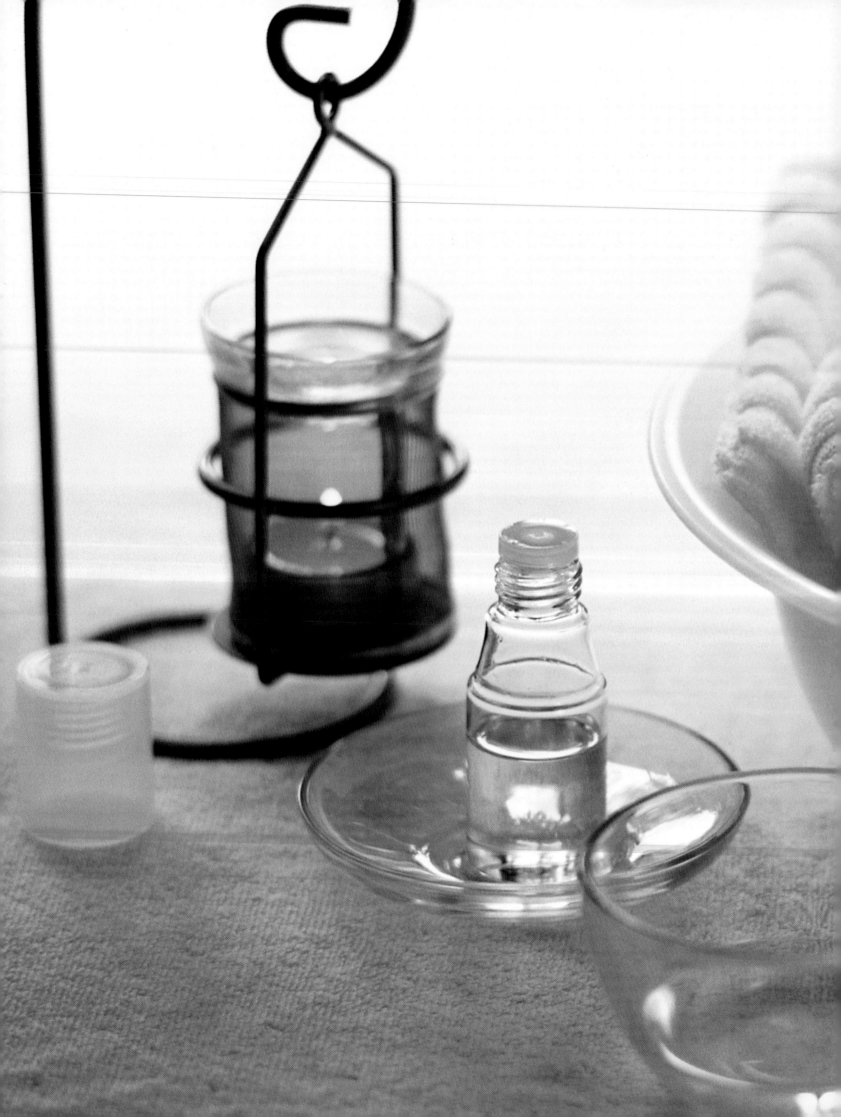

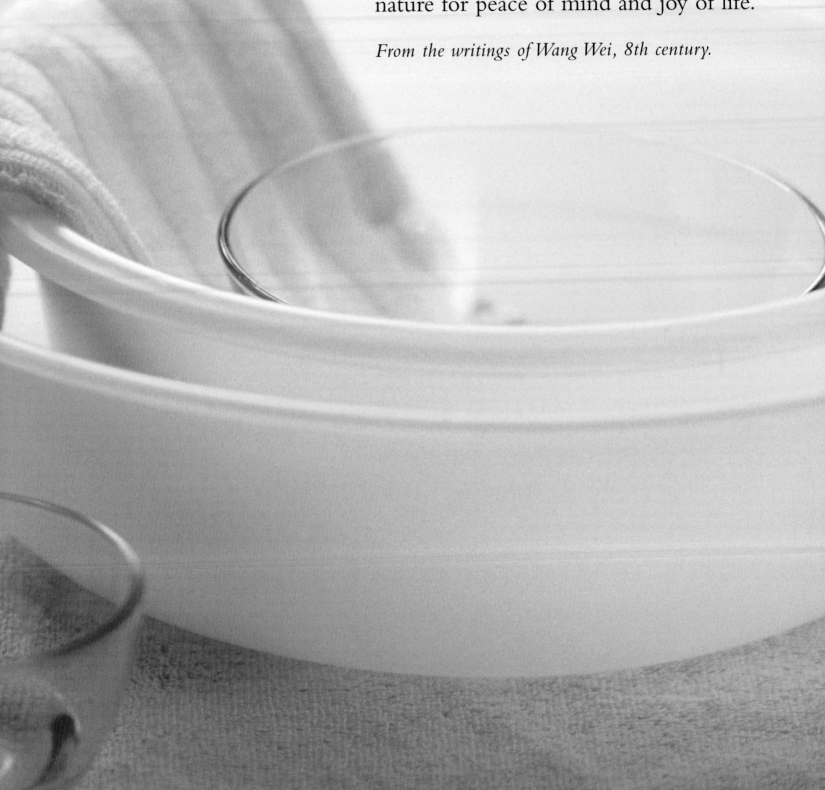

The Essential Oils

Look in the perfumes of flowers and of nature for peace of mind and joy of life.

From the writings of Wang Wei, 8th century.

The essential oils

Essential oils are powerful agents and all of them – even those nominated as safe – must be used in the correct amounts and for the conditions to which they are best suited. One or two pure essential oils, and most synthetic and adulterated ones, may cause irritation and skin sensitivity. The botanical varieties chosen for this book have been carefully selected from those which do not present this problem. However, these varieties are not always commonly available in the shops and appropriate cautions are included here for the sake of safety.

Except in emergencies, as in cases of burns, stings or wounds, essential oils should not be applied undiluted to the skin, but should be mixed first in a base carrier oil. Citrus oils are photosensitive and should not be used before sunbathing. If you are unsure about the suitability of an oil, always seek the advice of a qualified aromatherapist.

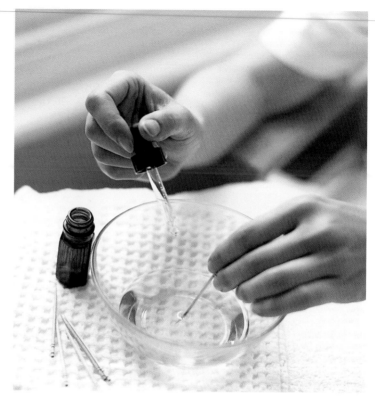

◁ **Prepare a compress for treatment at home by blending your favourite essential oils and adding them to water.**

▽ **Setting the scene at home will contribute to the benefits of aromatherapy. Choose a quiet part of the house and light candles to help you relax.**

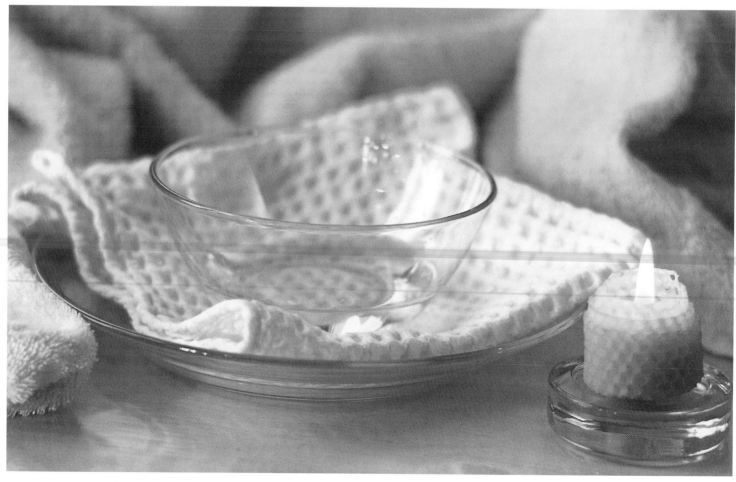

Boswellia carteri – frankincense
family *Burseraceae*

properties
analgesic, anti-infectious, antioxidant, anticatarrhal, antidepressive, anti-inflammatory, cicatrizant, energizing, expectorant, immunostimulant

These small trees, also known as olibanum, grow in north-east Africa and south-east Arabia. Cuts are made in the tree bark from which a white serum exudes, solidifying into "tear drops". When distilled, these produce a pale amber-green essential oil. Frankincense, an ancient aromatic product once considered as precious as gold, has been burnt in temples and used in religious ceremonies since Biblical times.

Frankincense is a gentle oil which is particularly useful for emotional problems, where it allays anger and irritability and soothes grief.

safety
• No known contraindications in normal aromatherapy use.

features in
Beauty and Well-being, The Reproductive Years, The Menopause, The Sunset Years.

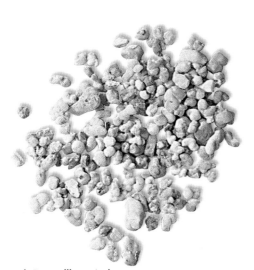

△ *Boswellia carteri* –
frankincense

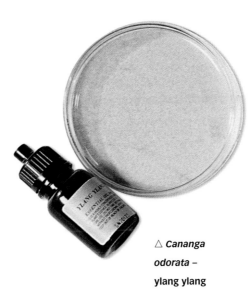

△ *Cananga odorata* –
ylang ylang

Cananga odorata – ylang ylang
family *Annonaceae*

properties
antidiabetic, antiseptic, antispasmodic, aphrodisiac, calming and sedative, hypotensive, general tonic, reproductive tonic

Ylang ylang trees, with their long, fluttering yellow-green flowers, are native to tropical Asia: ylang ylang is a Malay word meaning "flower of flowers". The blooms are picked early in the morning and steam-distilled to yield an oil with an exotic and heady aroma.

Widely reputed for its aphrodisiac qualities, ylang ylang is said to counter impotence and frigidity. It can help emotional problems such as irritability and fear; and is effective against introversion and shyness. Ylang ylang also helps to regulate cardiac and respiratory rhythm.

safety
• No known contraindications in normal aromatherapy use.
• Use in moderation. Excess can lead to nausea and headaches.

features in
The Teenage Years, Beauty and Well-being, The Menopause.

Cedrus atlantica – cedarwood
family *Pinaceae*

properties
antibacterial, antiseptic, cicatrizant, lipolytic, lymph tonic, mucolytic, stimulant

There are 20 or more species of the trees which yield an oil of cedar. This particular tree, the Atlas cedarwood, grows in the Atlas mountains of north Africa. The first oil extracted was used by the Egyptians for embalming. Most of the oil was taken from wood chippings left from making boxes and furniture (King Solomon used cedarwod extensively when building the temple at Jerusalem). Cedarwood oil is now obtained by steam distillation. It has a pleasant, sweet, woody aroma and can be used in a variety of ways.

Cedarwood is effective for oily skin and scalp disorders, and its antiseptic properties and cleansing aroma are beneficial to bronchial problems.

safety
• Unsuitable for pregnant women and small children.
• Should not be taken internally.

features in
The Teenage Years, Beauty and Well-being.

▽ *Cedrus atlantica* –
cedarwood

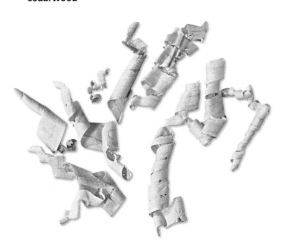

Chamaemelum nobile –
chamomile (Roman)
family *Asteraceae*

properties
antianaemic, anti-inflammatory, antineuralgic, antiparasitic, antispasmodic, calming and sedative, carminative, cicatrizant, digestive, emmenagogic, menstrual, vulnerary, stimulant, sudorific

Roman chamomile is native to the British Isles and is a small perennial with feathery leaves and daisy-like flowers. The essential oil is a pale blue-green colour because of the chamazulene content (see *Matricaria recutica* – German chamomile).

The oil is gentle, soothing and calming. It is suitable for children and babies for irritability, inability to sleep, hyperactivity and tantrums. Roman chamomile is also useful for a range of adult complaints, including rheumatic inflammation, indigestion and headaches.

safety
• No known contraindications in normal aromatherapy use.

features in
Beauty and Well-being, The Reproductive Years, The Menopause, The Sunset Years.

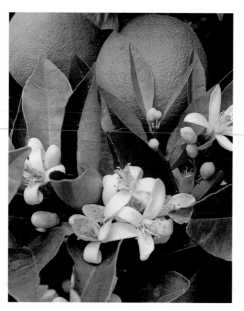

△ *Citrus aurantium* **var. *amara* – neroli**

Citrus aurantium var. *amara* –
neroli
family *Rutaceae*

properties
antidepressant, aphrodisiac, sedative, uplifting

Neroli oil is the distilled oil from the blossoms of the bitter orange tree. It has a soft, floral fragrance, and is the most costly of the orange oils.

Neroli is beneficial for the skin and helps improve its elasticity. It is good for scars, thread veins and the stretch marks of pregnancy and has a sedative and calming effect on the emotions.

safety
• No known contraindications in normal aromatherapy use.

features in
Beauty and Well-being, The Reproductive Years.

Citrus aurantium var. *amara* –
orange (bitter)
family *Rutaceae*

properties
anti-inflammatory, anticoagulant, calming, digestive, sedative, tonic

Oranges have a long tradition in both therapeutic and culinary use. A variety of essential oils are obtained from the fruit, flowers and leaves of both bitter (Seville) and sweet orange trees: neroli oil from the flowers, petitgrain from the leaves, and orange oil from the peel. Bitter orange is expressed from the peel of Seville oranges (most orange marmalades are also made from the peel of Seville oranges).

Bitter orange can be helpful for poor circulation, digestive problems and constipation. It has antidepressant qualities, and will promote positive thinking and cheerful feelings.

safety
• Photosensitizer. Do not expose the skin to sunlight or a sunbed for at least two hours after use.
• No known contraindications in normal aromatherapy use.

features in
The Reproductive Years, The Sunset Years.

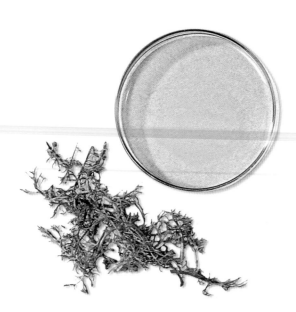

△ *Chamaemelum nobile* –
Roman chamomile

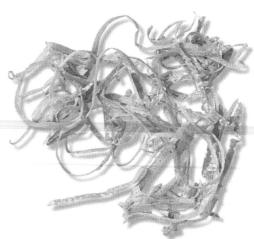

△ *Citrus aurantium* **var. *amara* –**
bitter orange

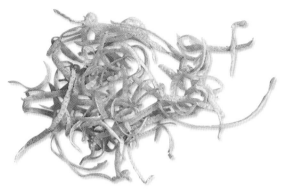

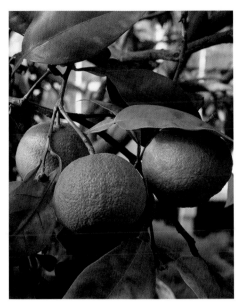

△ *Citrus aurantium* var. *amara* – petitgrain

△ *Citrus limon* – lemon

Citrus aurantium var. *amara* – petitgrain
family *Rutaceae*

properties
antibacterial, anti-infectious, anti-inflammatory, antispasmodic, calming and energizing

Taken from the leaves of the bitter orange tree, petitgrain's aroma is a cross between the delicate fragrance of neroli oil and the fresh aroma of bitter orange peel. A good petitgrain oil, distilled with some of the blossoms also, is often referred to as the "poor man's neroli" because of its enhanced aroma. Unlike the oil from the fruit, which is expressed, petitgrain oil is obtained by distillation.

Petitgrain is balancing to the nervous system and is recommended for infected skin problems. Emotionally, it can help with anger and panic.

safety
• No known contraindications in normal aromatherapy use.

features in
The Teenage Years.

Citrus bergamia – bergamot
family *Rutaceae*

properties
antibacterial, anti-infectious, antiseptic, antispasmodic, antiviral, calming and sedative, cicatrizant, tonic, stomachic

The main area of bergamot production is southern Italy, although it is also grown on the Ivory Coast. The greenish essential oil is expressed from the peel of this bitter, inedible citrus fruit, which in Cyprus is often crystallized and eaten with a cup of tea. Traditionally, bergamot is a principal ingredient in eau-de-cologne because of its refreshing aroma, and is famous for its use as the flavouring in Earl Grey tea.

Bergamot is useful both in the treatment of digestive problems, such as colic, spasm and sluggish digestion, and for calming emotional states, such as agitation and severe mood swings. It is effective on cold sores but use with extreme caution if in strong sunlight.

safety
• Photosensitizer. Do not expose the skin to sunlight or a sunbed until at least two hours after using.
• Bergapten-free bergamot is an adulterated oil and should not be substituted for the whole essential oil. If not going into the sun, bergamot can be used in the same way as any other oil without risk.

features in
Beauty and Well-being, The Sunset Years.

▷ *Citrus bergamia* – bergamot

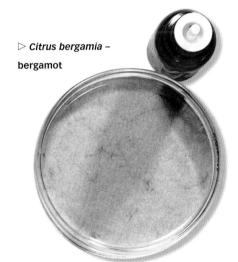

Citrus limon – lemon
family *Rutaceae*

properties
antianaemic, antibacterial, anticoagulant, antifungal, anti-infectious, anti-inflammatory, antisclerotic, antiseptic, antispasmodic, antiviral, calming, carminative, digestive, diuretic, expectorant, immunostimulant, litholytic, phlebotonic, stomachic

Lemon juice and peel are widely used in cooking, and the essential oil is expressed from the peel of fruit not sprayed with harmful chemicals. Natural waxes in the oil may appear if it is kept at too low a temperature, but this does not detract from its quality or effectiveness.

Oil of lemon is an underestimated and extremely useful oil. It has an anti-infectious and expectorant effect on the respiratory airways and can help to eliminate the toxins which cause arthritic pain. It is also good for greasy skin. The clean, lively scent can lift the spirits, dispel sluggishness and indecision and relieve depression. Oil of lemon can also help to dispel fear and apathy.

safety
• Photosensitizer. Do not expose the skin to sunlight or a sunbed for two hours after using.

features in
The Teenage Years, Beauty and Well-being, The Reproductive Years, The Sunset Years.

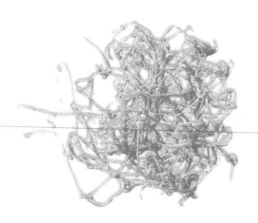

△ *Citrus paradis* –

grapefruit

Citrus paradis – grapefruit
family *Rutaceae*

properties
antiseptic, aperitif, digestive, diuretic

Originating in tropical Asia and the West Indies, the grapefruit tree is now cultivated mainly in North and South America. The yellow oil, produced mainly in California, is obtained by expression of the peel and has a sweet, citrus aroma.

It is effective in caring for oily skin and acne, and regular use twice daily is helpful for cellulite, water retention and obesity. Its antiseptic property is particularly useful in a vapourizer to disinfect the air of a sickroom. It is useful to add a little (4 drops per litre) to spring water when travelling to help prevent digestive problems.

safety
• No known contraindications in normal aromatherapy use.

features in
The Teenage Years, Beauty and Well-being, The Sunset Years.

Citrus reticulata – mandarin
family *Rutaceae*

properties
antifungal, antispasmodic, calming, digestive

The mandarin orange tree originates in China, and its fruit was named after the Chinese Mandarins. The fruit of the mandarin tree is very similar to the tangerine and oils from both fruits may be sold as mandarin. The essential oil is expressed from the peel.

Mandarin oil has digestive properties, and is excellent for treating both adults and children with indigestion, stomach pains and constipation. It can be very useful for over-excitement, stress and insomnia. It is often popular with children because of its gentle action and familiar orangey aroma.

safety
• No known contraindications in normal aromatherapy use.

features in
The Reproductive Years, The Sunset Years.

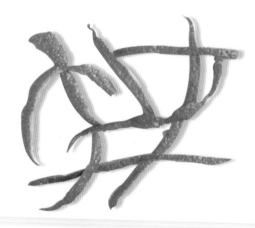

△ *Citrus reticulata* –

mandarin

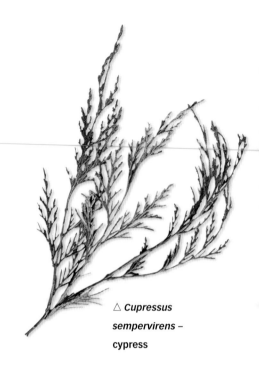

△ *Cupressus*

sempervirens –

cypress

Cupressus sempervirens – cypress
family *Cupressaceae*

properties
antibacterial, anti-infectious, antispasmodic, antisudorific, antitussive, astringent, calming, deodorant, diuretic, hormone-like, neurotonic, phlebotonic, styptic

Cypress oil is distilled from the leaves, cones and twigs of the cypress tree. *Sempervirens* is Latin for evergreen, and the resinous wood of this ancient tree has long been used as an aromatic.

The astringent action of cypress oil helps to regulate the production of sebum, reduce perspiration (even of the feet) and to staunch bleeding. It is reputed to help calm the mind where grief is present, and to induce sleep.

safety
• No known contraindications in normal aromatherapy use.

features in
Beauty and Well-being, The Reproductive Years, The Menopause, The Sunset Years.

Eucalyptus smithii – eucalyptus
family *Myrtaceae*

properties
analgesic, anticatarrhal, anti-infectious, antiviral, balancing, decongestant, digestive stimulant, expectorant, prophylactic

Known as gully gum, this tree is native to Australia. The oil distilled from its leaves is equally beneficial to, and much gentler than, the more common *Eucalyptus globulus*, or blue gum, which needs care in use. Because of its gentle action, gully gum eucalyptus is ideal for children; its aroma is also not as piercing as blue gum eucalyptus, which is usually rectified to increase its cineole content.

Eucalyptus is good for muscular pain and is effective against coughs and colds, both as a preventive and as a remedy. *E. smithii* oil has great synergistic power.

safety
- No known contraindications in normal aromatherapy use.
- Keep to the recommended dilution when using as an inhalant for children.

features in:
Beauty and Well-being, The Reproductive Years, The Sunset Years.

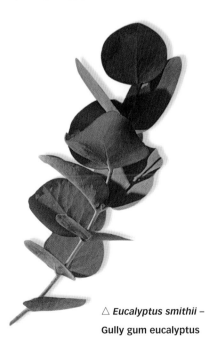

△ *Eucalyptus smithii* –
Gully gum eucalyptus

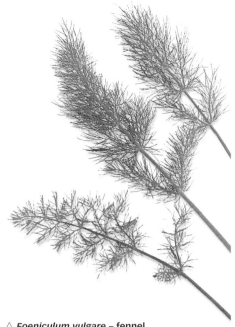

△ *Foeniculum vulgare* – fennel

Foeniculum vulgare – fennel
family *Apiaceae* (or *Umbelliferae*)

properties
analgesic, antibacterial, antifungal, anti-inflammatory, antiseptic, antispasmodic, cardiotonic, carminative, decongestant, digestive, diuretic, emmenagogic, lactogenic, laxative, litholytic, oestrogen-like, respiratory tonic

Fennel is widely grown in the Mediterranean area and the essential oil is distilled from its seeds. The delicate flower heads of all this family resemble umbrellas, as indicated by the original family name, *Umbelliferae*.

Fennel is recommended for lack of breast milk and because it is oestrogen-like, it can be valuable for PMS, the menopause and ovary problems. It will also work efficiently as a diuretic.

safety
- Safe in normal aromatherapy amounts.
- Should not be used during pregnancy before the seventh month.

features in
Beauty and Well-being, The Reproductive Years.

Juniperus communis – juniper
family *Cupressaceae*

properties
analgesic, antidiabetic, antiseptic, depurative, digestive tonic, diuretic, litholytic, sleep-inducing

The juniper tree is a small evergreen from the same family as cypress. The essential oil, distilled from the dried ripe berries (and sometimes the twigs and leaves), has a sweet fragrant aroma. Take care when buying juniper oil, as the berries are used to flavour gin and the residue is often distilled to produce a poor quality essential oil. Even genuine juniper oil can be frequently adulterated.

Juniper oil has a strong diuretic action which is useful for treating cystitis, water retention and cellulite. It has a cleansing, detoxifying action on the skin, and is useful for oily skin problems, such as acne. It is especially good for feelings of guilt and jealousy, and for giving strength when feeling emotionally drained.

safety
- No known contraindications in normal aromatherapy use.
- May be neurotoxic if used without due care and attention.

features in
The Teenage Years, Beauty and Well-being, The Reproductive Years, The Menopause.

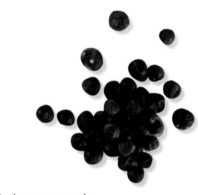

△ *Juniperus communis* –
juniper

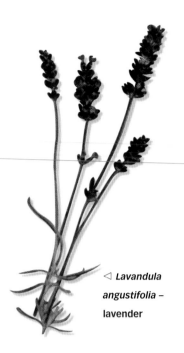

◁ *Lavandula angustifolia* – lavender

Lavandula angustifolia – lavender
family *Lamiaceae*

properties
analgesic, antibacterial, antifungal, anti-inflammatory, antiseptic, antispasmodic, calming and sedative, cardiotonic, carminative, cicatrizant, emmenagogic, hypotensive, tonic

Lavender is the most widely used aromatherapy oil. It is obtained from the plant's flowering tops, and grows wild throughout the Mediterranean region, although it is now cultivated worldwide. In spite of this, it is not easy to find a quality oil. Lavandin, a cheaper oil from a hybrid plant, is often substituted for true lavender.

Lavender is a skin rejuvenator, and helps to normalize both dry and greasy skins. It works in combination with other oils to alleviate arthritis and rheumatism, psoriasis and eczema. It aids sleep, relieves tension headaches, and is good for calming nerves, lifting depression, relieving anger, and soothing fear and grief.

safety
• No known contraindications in normal aromatherapy use.

features in
The Teenage Years, Beauty and Well-being, The Reproductive Years, The Menopause, The Sunset Years.

Matricaria recutica – chamomile, German
family *Asteraceae*

properties
antiallergic, antifungal, anti-inflammatory, antispasmodic, cicatrizant, decongestant, digestive tonic, hormone-like

German chamomile, an annual herb, grows naturally in Europe and its small white flowers are widely used in teas and infusions to aid relaxation and induce sleep. When the flowers are distilled a deep blue oil is produced. The blue colour is produced by the presence of chamazulene, a chemical not present in the plant but formed during the distillation process.

Chamazulene, in synergy with the other components of the oil, is a strong anti-inflammatory agent, which is especially useful for skin problems (particularly irritated skin) and rheumatism, when a compress is most effective. The oil is recommended for premenstrual syndrome, and for calming anger and agitated emotional states.

safety
• No known contraindications in normal aromatherapy use.

features in
Beauty and Well-being, The Reproductive Years, The Sunset Years.

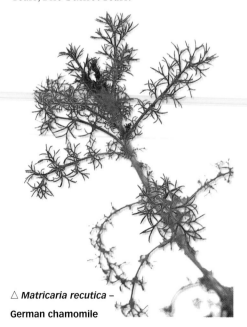

△ *Matricaria recutica* – German chamomile

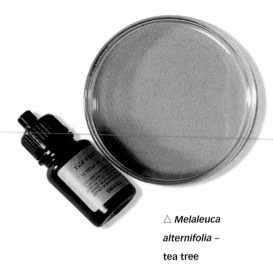

△ *Melaleuca alternifolia* – tea tree

Melaleuca alternifolia – tea tree
family *Myrtaceae*

properties
analgesic, antibacterial, antifungal, anti-infectious, anti-inflammatory, antiparasitic, antiviral, immunostimulant, neurotonic, phlebotonic

The tea tree plant is native to Australia. Traditionally, a type of herbal tea is prepared from its leaves, and the oil has long been recognized by the Australian Aborigines for its powerful medicinal properties.

Essential oil of tea tree has strong antiseptic properties with a matching aroma, and has excellent antimicrobial and antifungal action. It is a powerful stimulant to the immune system. The unadulterated essential oil has been found to be non-toxic and non-irritating to the skin, and is one of the few essential oils that can be applied directly and undiluted on the skin and all mucous surfaces. The antifungal activity of tea tree oil is much used against *Candida albicans*. It is also effective against some viruses, such as enteritis.

safety
• No known contraindications in normal aromatherapy use.

features in
The Teenage Years, Beauty and Well-being.

Melaleuca viridiflora – niaouli
family *Myrtaceae*

properties
analgesic, antibacterial, anticatarrhal, anti-infectious, anti-inflammatory, antiparasitic, antipruritic, antirheumatic, antiseptic, antiviral, digestive, expectorant, febrifuge, hormone-like, hypotensive, immunostimulant, litholytic, phlebotonic, skin tonic

Niaouli trees originate from the region of Gomene in the South Pacific island of New Caledonia, hence "gomenol" became an alternative name. The trees are large with a bushy foliage and yellow flowers. The steam-distilled leaves and young stems yield an essential oil, which has a eucalyptus-type aroma. The majority of the oil is produced in Australia and Tasmania and very little is exported, making the genuine oil hard to find.

Niaouli is useful for a range of problems experienced by women. It is also a powerful antiseptic and anti-inflammatory agent, and is effective for respiratory problems, such as bronchitis and colds. Its properties suggest it will help against grief and anger.

safety
• No known contraindications, but pregnant women and children should use with care.

features in
Beauty and Well-being, The Reproductive Years, The Sunset Years.

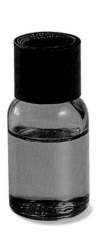

◁ *Melaleuca viridiflora – niaouli*

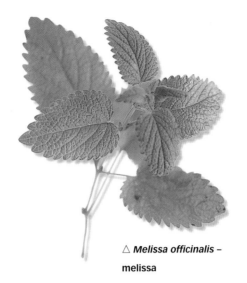

△ *Melissa officinalis – melissa*

Melissa officinalis – melissa
family *Lamiaceae*

properties
anti-inflammatory, antispasmodic, antiviral, calming and sedative, choleretic, digestive, hypotensive, sedative, capillary dilator

Melissa, also known as lemon balm, is a small herb with tiny, white flowers originating from southern Europe. A daily drink of tea prepared from the fresh leaves is supposed to encourage longevity. The distilled yield from the leaves is tiny, making it a very expensive oil. Much of the melissa oil sold commercially is blended with cheaper essential oils and achieves a similar aroma.

Melissa's sedative action relieves headaches and insomnia and is particularly beneficial for a problematic menstrual cycle. It is also a tonic for the heart, calming the turbulent emotions of grief and anger and helping to relieve fear.

safety
• Photosensitizer. Do not expose the skin to sunlight or a sunbed for two hours after using.
• It is difficult to obtain pure melissa oil, and many fakes contain skin irritants.
• No known contraindications in normal aromatherapy use.

features in
Beauty and Well-being, The Reproductive Years, The Sunset Years.

Mentha piperita – peppermint
family *Lamiaceae*

properties
analgesic, antibacterial, antifungal, anti-inflammatory, antimigraine, antilactogenic, antipyretic, antispasmodic, antiviral, carminative, decongestant, digestive, expectorant, liver stimulant, hormone-like, hypotensive, insect repellent, mucolytic, neurotonic, reproductive stimulant, soothing, uterotonic

The peppermint plant has dark green leaves from which its essential oil is distilled. The oil has a strong, refreshing aroma and is used extensively in the food and pharmaceutical industries, particularly for toothpaste, chewing gum and drinks.

Peppermint is renowned not only for its beneficial effect with digestive problems, such as indigestion, nausea, travel sickness, and diarrhoea, but also for respiratory problems. It can help to clear congestion or catarrh and is useful for bronchitis, bronchial asthma, sinusitis and colds. It helps to clear the mind, and will aid concentration and overcome mental fatigue and depression. It is also useful against anger, guilt and apathy. This is a good essential oil to keep to hand in the first aid cabinet.

safety
• Use sparingly and keep to recommended dilution.
• May counteract homeopathic remedies.

features in
Beauty and Well-being, The Reproductive Years, The Menopause, The Sunset Years.

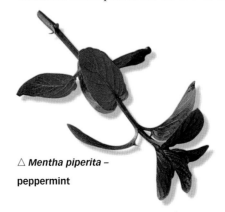

△ *Mentha piperita – peppermint*

Ocimum basilicum var. *album* – basil
family *Lamiaceae*

properties
analgesic, antibacterial, antifungal, anti-inflammatory, antiseptic, antispasmodic, antiviral, cardiotonic, carminative, digestive tonic, nervous system regulator, neurotonic, reproductive decongestant

Basil oil has a distinctive aroma and is distilled from the whole plant. Several varieties of basil, with different chemical composition, grow in warm Mediterranean climes (especially France and Italy), with leaves that vary in both size and colour, from green to a deep purplish red. The preferred variety for aromatherapy is *album*, as it is not likely to have a neurotoxic effect.

Basil is known mainly for its effect on the nervous system. It is a good tonic and stimulant and is helpful in coping with unwanted emotions, such as fear and jealousy. Its analgesic property makes it useful in cases of arthritis. It is also good for muscle cramp. Basil is an effective insect repellent, particularly against house flies and mosquitoes.

safety
• No known contraindications in normal aromatherapy use.
• May be neurotoxic if used without due care and attention.

features in
Beauty and Well-being, The Reproductive Years, The Menopause, The Sunset Years.

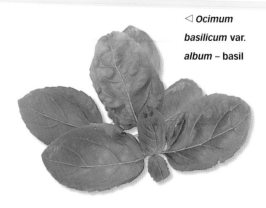

◁ *Ocimum basilicum* var. *album* – basil

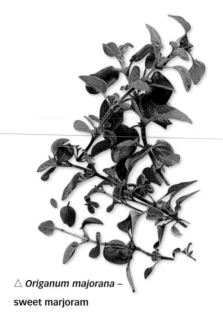

△ *Origanum majorana* – sweet marjoram

Origanum majorana – *sweet* marjoram
family *Lamiaceae*

properties
analgesic, antibacterial, anti-infectious, antispasmodic, calming, digestive stimulant, diuretic, expectorant, hormone-like, hypotensive, neurotonic, respiratory tonic, stomachic, vasodilator

Sweet marjoram is a popular culinary herb and has a reputation for promoting long life. The plant grows in the Mediterranean regions and has tiny, white or pink flowers: the oil is distilled from the plant's leaves and flowers. Sweet marjoram should not be confused with the sharp-smelling Spanish marjoram (*Thymus mastichina*), which is a species of thyme.

Sweet marjoram has been shown to be antiviral and is useful for cold sores. It can ease tension and irritability, lift headaches (especially those connected with menstruation) and promote sleep. It is useful for grief and anger, and its ability to calm and uplift makes it useful to combat moodiness.

safety
• No known contraindications in normal aromatherapy use.

features in
Beauty and Well-being, The Reproductive Years, The Menopause, The Sunset Years.

Pelargonium graveolens – geranium
family *Geraniaceae*

properties
analgesic, antibacterial, antidiabetic, antifungal, anti-infectious, anti-inflammatory, antiseptic, antispasmodic, astringent, cicatrizant, decongestant, digestive stimulant, haemostatic, styptic, insect repellent, phlebotonic, relaxant

The geranium plant is cultivated in Egypt, Morocco, the Reunion Islands and China. The oil is distilled from the aromatic leaves, the aroma of which depends on the variety of the plant and where it is grown. Some geranium oils have a definite rose-like smell and are often referred to as rose geranium. More correctly, rose geranium is when a tiny percentage of rose otto is added to the geranium oil.

Geranium will reduce inflammation and is good for acne, herpes, diarrhoea and varicose veins. It is also a relaxant, and will help grief and anger. It is useful for general moodiness and to balance the mood swings associated with PMS.

safety
• No known contraindications in normal aromatherapy use.

features in
The Teenage Years, Beauty and Well-being, The Reproductive Years, The Menopause, The Sunset Years.

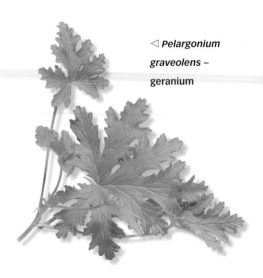

◁ *Pelargonium graveolens* – geranium

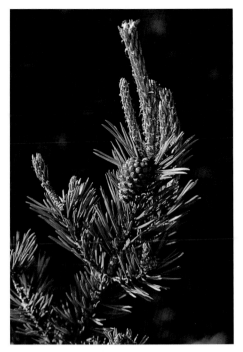
△ *Pinus sylvestris* – pine

Pinus sylvestris – pine
family *Pinaceae*

properties
analgesic, antibacterial, antifungal, anti-infectious, anti-inflammatory, antisudorific, balsamic, decongestant, expectorant, hormone-like, hypotensive, litholytic, neurotonic, rubefacient

Pine-needle essential oil has a warm, resin-like aroma and is distilled from the Scots-pine tree, which grows widely throughout Europe and Russia.

Pine is an excellent disinfectant and air-freshener: when dispersed in the air, its antiseptic qualities help to prevent the spread of infections. It is recommended for respiratory tract infections and hay fever, while its anti-inflammatory action makes it useful for cystitis and rheumatism. Pine is an excellent pick-me-up for general debility and lack of energy, and is said to dispel melancholy and pessimism.

safety
• No known contraindications in normal aromatherapy use.

features in
Beauty and Well-being, The Reproductive Years, The Menopause, The Sunset Years.

Pogostemon patchouli – patchouli
family *Lamiaceae*

properties
antifungal, anti-infectious, anti-inflammatory, aphrodisiac, cicatrizant, decongestant, immunostimulant, insect repellent, phlebotonic

The plant grows mainly in East Asia and its essential oil has a soft, balsamic aroma. The leaves are cut every few months as the newest ones yield the most oil. Patchouli oil improves with age and has a musty, exotic aroma that is very penetrating.

Patchouli is particularly valuable for broken, chapped and cracked skin, as well as inflamed skin, eczema and acne. It promotes the growth of new skin cells, which makes it helpful in reducing scar tissue. It is beneficial against haemorrhoids and varicose veins. It has a sedative effect on the emotions; its anti-inflammatory property helps calm anger and its antifungal property is useful for jealousy. It is said to help soothe an overactive mind.

safety
• No known contraindications in normal aromatherapy use.

features in
Beauty and Well-being, The Reproductive Years.

▷ *Pogostemon patchouli* – **patchouli**

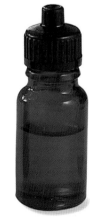

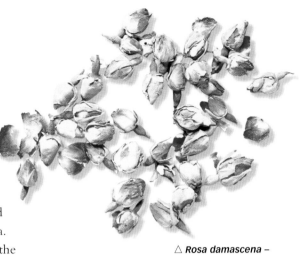
△ *Rosa damascena* – rose otto

Rosa damascena – rose otto
family *Rosaceae*

properties
antibacterial, anti-infectious, anti-inflammatory, astringent, cicatrizant, neurotonic, sexual tonic, styptic

The much-prized rose otto, also known as attar of roses, is distilled from the deep pink rose petals of this flowering shrub. The genuine, pure oil is extremely expensive as the petals contain very little oil. Roses for distillation are cultivated chiefly in Bulgaria, Turkey and Morocco. Rose absolute is extracted from the petals by a different process, and is a cheaper oil.

Rose otto has been favoured by women through the ages for its gentle action and fragrant aroma. It is said that rose otto balances the hormones and that it is helpful for irregular periods. Rose soothes the skin, lifts depression, and calms inflamed emotions, promoting feelings of happiness and well-being.

safety
• No known contraindications in normal aromatherapy use.

features in
Beauty and Well-being, The Reptroductive Years, The Menopause.

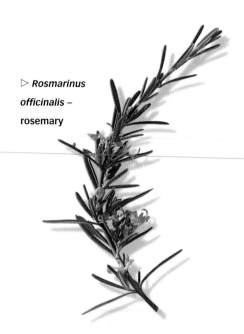

▷ *Rosmarinus officinalis –* rosemary

Rosmarinus officinalis – rosemary
family *Lamiaceae*

properties
analgesic, antibacterial, antifungal, anti-infectious, anti-inflammatory, antispasmodic, antitussive, antiviral, cardiotonic, carminative, choleretic, cicatrizant, venous decongestant, detoxicant, digestive, diuretic, emmenagogic, hyperglycaemic, blood pressure regulator, litholytic, cholesterol-reducing, mucolytic, neuromuscular effect, neurotonic, sexual tonic, stimulant

Native to the Mediterranean region, rosemary has a long history of culinary and medicinal use. This oil, with an impressive list of helpful properties, is obtained from the pale-blue flowers of the aromatic plant.

Rosemary is helpful for respiratory problems, arthritis, congestive headaches and constipation. It is also a tonic for the liver. This oil stimulates both body and mind. It lifts depression, clears the mind, and is an excellent memory aid.

safety
No known contraindications in normal aromatherapy use.

features in
The Teenage Years, Beauty and Well-being, The Reproductive Years, The Menopause, The Sunset Years.

Salvia sclarea – clary sage
family *Lamiaceae*

properties
antifungal, anti-infectious, antispasmodic, antisudorific, decongestant, detoxicant, oestrogen-like, neurotonic, phlebotonic, regenerative

The strong smelling essential oil of clary sage is distilled from the dried clary sage plant and is used in eau-de-cologne, lavender water, muscatel wines and vermouth. It should not be confused with sage oil and is not a substitute for it.

Clary sage is excellent for all menstrual complications; its oestrogen-like qualities make it good for hormonal problems. It encourages menstruation and is useful for the hot flushes of the menopause. Clary sage is helpful for depression and fear, and during general convalescence.

Safety
• No known contraindications in normal aromatherapy use.
• Prolonged inhalation may cause drowsiness.
• Avoid alcohol consumption for a few hours before or after use.

features in
The Teenage Years, Beauty and Well-being, The Reproductive Years, The Menopause, The Sunset Years.

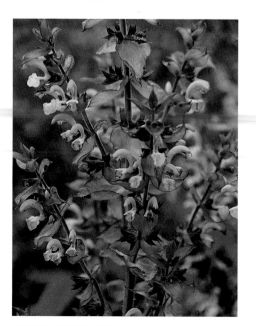

△ *Salvia sclarea –* clary sage

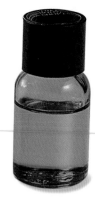

▷ *Santalum album –* sandalwood

Santalum album – sandalwood
family *Santalaceae*

properties
anti-infectious, astringent, cardiotonic, decongestant, diuretic, moisturizing, nerve relaxant, sedative, tonic

The sandalwood tree is native to India, and its cultivation is controlled by the government of that country – for each tree felled, another is planted. The offcuts and wood chips from the sandalwood furniture industry in India, together with the tree roots, are distilled to obtain the essential oil. The sweet, woody aroma of the oil has a soft and therapeutic effect.

Sandalwood, although a gentle oil, is important in the treatment of genito-urinary infections, especially cystisis. It is used for its effect on the digestive system, relieving heartburn and nausea, including morning sickness. It has been found to benefit both acne and dry skin (including dry eczema), as well as being useful for haemorrhoids and varicose veins. Its tonic properties are thought to be helpful in cases of impotence. Sandalwood can also be useful against fear.

Safety
• No known contraindications in normal aromatherapy use.

features in
The Teenage Years, Beauty and Well-being, The Reproductive Years, The Menopause, The Sunset Years.

Thymus vulgaris – thyme, sweet
family *Lamiaceae*

properties
antifungal, anti-infectious, anti-inflammatory, antiseptic, antispasmodic, antiviral, diuretic, immunostimulant, neurotonic, sexual tonic, uterotonic

Thyme is native to the Mediterranean region and is a well-known culinary herb. The essential oil is distilled from its leaves and tiny purplish flowers. There are many different varieties of thyme oil, some of which need careful handling. The alcohol chemotypes of thyme (linalool and geraniol) are the safest for general use.

Sweet thyme is useful for respiratory problems, infections, and digestive complaints. It is especially helpful for insomnia of nervous origin. Sweet thyme is a safe, uterotonic oil to use towards the end of pregnancy and during labour, and it is known to facilitate delivery.

safety
• No known contraindications in normal aromatherapy use.

features in
Beauty and Well-being, The Menopause.

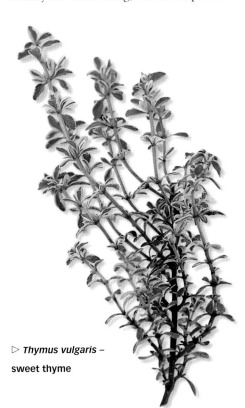

▷ *Thymus vulgaris –*
sweet thyme

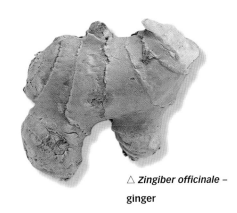

△ *Zingiber officinale –*
ginger

Zingiber officinale – ginger
family *Zingiberaceae*

properties
analgesic, anticatarrhal, carminative, digestive stimulant, expectorant, general tonic, sexual tonic, stomachic

This perennial herb is native to the tropical parts of Asia. The root, which is used in cooking, is renowned for its heat and for its digestive properties. Its yellow oil is distilled from the roots and, although it has a spicy aroma, the heat does not come through into the essential oil during distillation.

Ginger essential oil has properties which alleviate most digestive problems, including flatulence, constipation, nausea and loss of appetite. Its ability to dull pain is beneficial to muscular pain and sciatica, while its tonic properties are useful for emotions like fear and apathy, and will also help to draw out a reticent, withdrawn personality.

safety
• No known contraindications in normal aromatherapy use.

features in
The Reproductive Years, The Sunset Years.

Special essential oils

Myristica fragrans – nutmeg
Pimpinella anisum – aniseed
Salvia officinalis – sage
Syzygium aromaticum – clove bud

There are some highly beneficial, but very powerful oils which are recommended in this book for special use only. These are used in pregnancy to facilitate delivery. However, their use is not advised without training in aromatherapy or aromatic medicine.

safety
• These oils must only be used in the manner and amounts advised.
• Always seek advice from a qualified aromatherapist before home use.

featured in
Pregnancy.

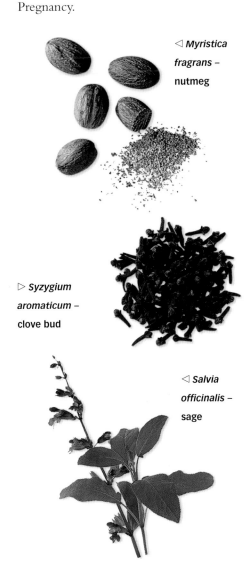

◁ *Myristica fragrans –*
nutmeg

▷ *Syzygium aromaticum –*
clove bud

◁ *Salvia officinalis –*
sage

Aromatherapy Techniques

Physicians might…make greater use of scents than they do, for I have often noticed that they cause changes in me, and act on my spirits.

From Essay on Smell, Michel Eyquem de Montaigne, 1533–1592.

Using inhalations and baths

Essential oils are rarely used in their original, concentrated form but are always taken into the body via a carrier substance. This can be anything which takes the oils into the body: air, water, vegetable oils, lotions and creams are all carriers.

inhalation

When we breathe in the fragrance of an essential oil, some of its molecules travel to the lungs, pass through the lining and into the bloodstream, where they travel around the body. Other molecules take an upward route to the brain, which receives a healing message – to relax or energize, for example – and transmits the appropriate signal along the nerve channels of the body.

Inhalation is the quickest way for oils to enter the body, and is the most effective way to deal with fragile emotions, and negative states of mind such as stress and depression. It is very useful for respiratory conditions, especially those that may present an emergency situation, such as bronchitis or asthma Although essential oils may be inhaled directly from the bottle, other methods are preferred.

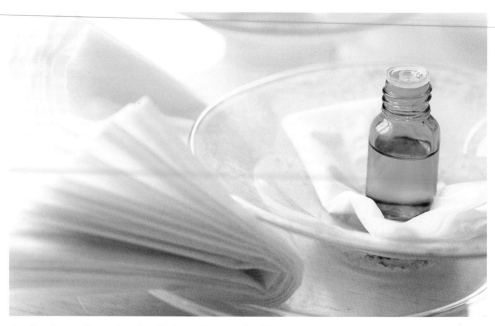

△ **A few drops of lavender oil, added to a tissue and sniffed throughout the day, can relieve headaches.**

the hands

This method is useful for emergencies. Put one drop of essential oil into your palm and rub your hands briefly together. Now cup your hands over your nose, avoiding the eye area, and take a deep breath.

a tissue

Place a few drops of essential oil on to a tissue and take three deep breaths. The tissue can then be placed on your pillow or inside your shirt, so that you will continue to benefit from the oil's aroma.

steam inhalation

Fill a basin with hot water and add no more than 2–3 drops (use 1–2 drops for children and the elderly) of essential oil. Keeping your eyes closed to protect them from the powerful vapours, lower your head over the bowl and breathe in deeply.

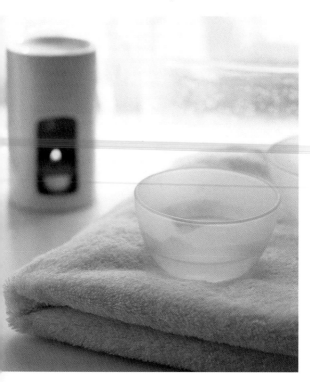

◁ **Using an oil burner is a popular way of vaporizing essential oils. Keep enough water in the top to stop it drying out.**

▷ **A steam inhalation using eucalyptus oil can help to relieve head colds and sinus congestion.**

a vaporizer

This is one of the most popular methods of all for oil inhalation. Electric vaporizers are available, and are the safest types to use. Night-light vaporizers (or oil burners) are inexpensive and readily available in different sizes and designs. The basic model involves a night-light candle standing under a tiny

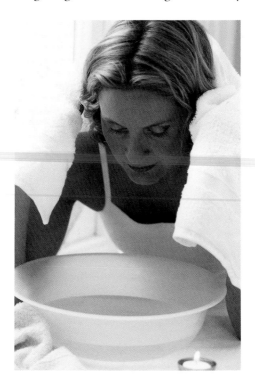

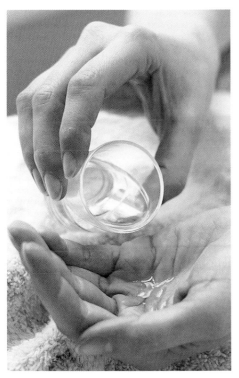

△ **Dry skin will benefit from an essential oil mix: it is best massaged on to your body after a bath.**

cup filled with water, to which a few drops of oil are added. Keep the vaporizer out of the reach of children and pets. Top up the water and add more oils as necessary.

Use a vaporizer to keep infections at bay, to relax after a stressful day, or to set the mood for a party or a romantic evening. The number of oil drops is not critical and really depends on the size of the room.

safety
• The quantities of essential oils given above for inhalations are suitable for children and the elderly unless otherwise stated.

bathing
Essential oils do not dissolve well in water, and it is important that the molecules are evenly distributed. Bathing can enhance the effects of essential oils: the oils are not only absorbed through the skin but their aroma is also inhaled. There are several ways to enjoy bathing with essential oils.

bath
Run the water in the bath to a comfortable temperature. Next, add 6-8 drops of oil, then swish the water thoroughly to disperse

▷ **Pamper yourself and unwind with a relaxing aromatherapy bath at the end of a tiring day.**

the oil. Sit in the bath, and for maximum benefit, stay in the water for at least ten minutes to allow the oil to penetrate your skin and to enjoy the benefits of its aroma.

If you prefer, the oils can be mixed with 15 ml/1 tbsp dairy cream or honey before being added to the bath. This will help to disperse the oils. Alternatively, you can mix the oils into powdered milk, adding water to make a paste, before adding the mixture to the bath water. Bath oil prepared from vegetable oil and mixed with essential oils is fine for dry skin, but will feel greasy on normal skins.

foot and hand bath
For sprains, localized swelling, bruising, or similar general discomforts, ten minutes in a foot or hand bath containing 6-8 drops of your chosen oils will bring welcome relief. Remember to keep a kettle of warm water nearby to add to the water in the bowl before it cools too much for comfort.

sitz-bath
For vaginal thrush, a sitz-bath with essential oils is an effective treatment. Fill a large bowl one-third full with warm water and add 3-4 drops of your chosen oil. Sit in the bath for ten minutes.

showers
It is not as easy to benefit from essential oils in the shower. However, you can add some oils to your shower gel or put some on to a sponge. Rub this over your body in the shower, or before you get into it. Make the most of the aroma, breathing deeply and rubbing with your sponge or hands while slowly rinsing. If you wash off the oils too quickly, you won't feel the benefit. Finish with a body lotion mixed with an oil.

safety
• For children and the elderly the essential oil quantities should be halved.

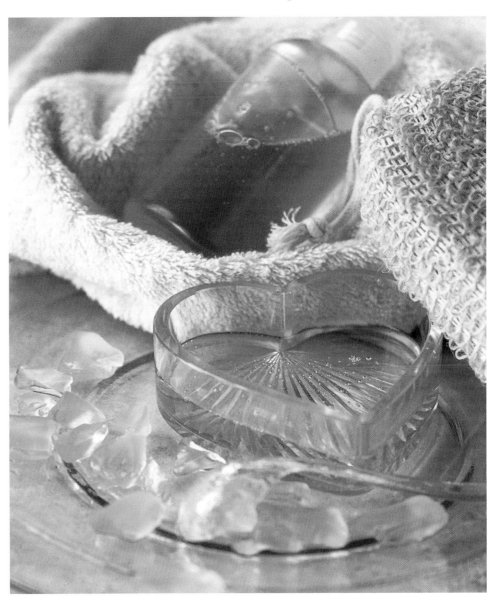

Using compresses, gargles and drinks

Further effective ways of carrying essential oils into the body, using water as the carrier, are with compresses, gargles, mouthwashes and drinks. For the latter, it is important that the essential oils used, and the number of drops, are exactly as recommended.

compresses

A compress brings effective relief in cases such as insect bites, arthritic joints, period or stomach pain, headache, sprains and varicose veins. Use a cold compress if there is inflammation and/or heat, and a warm compress if there is pain or a dull ache.

To make the compress, you need a piece of clean material and a container of water. Soft cotton or linen are the best materials to

▽ **A compress is a simple way to use essential oils, and the result can be very soothing.**

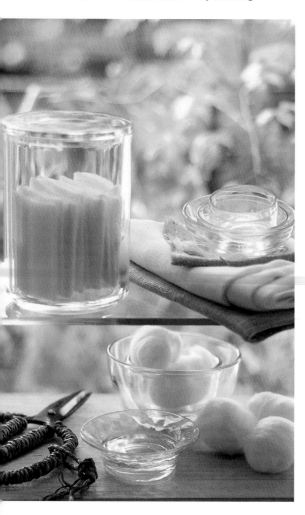

use. The container should be big enough to hold just enough water to soak into the compress: for example, an egg cup will be big enough for a finger compress, and a small bowl is suitable for an abdomen compress. Add your chosen essential oils to the water: 2 drops of oil is enough for a finger compress, and up to 8 drops of oil is enough for larger body compresses.

Stir the water in the container to disperse the essential oils, then gently lower the compress material on top to allow it to absorb the oils. When the material is wet, squeeze it lightly, position it on the area to be treated, and cover with cling film (plastic wrap) to hold it firmly in place.

For a cold compress, place a sealed, plastic bag of frozen peas or crushed ice cubes over the treatment area and hold in place. For a warm compress, wrap a strip of material such as a scarf, thermal garment or a small towel around the cling film. To keep a compress in place on an arm or leg, an old sock or pair of tights is ideal. Leave the compress in place for at least an hour, or overnight for a septic wound.

gargles and mouthwashes

For sore throats, voice loss and colds which may go on to the chest, gargling with one or more essential oils can be very helpful. Put 2–3 drops of antibacterial essential oils into a glass and half-fill with water. A drop of a soothing oil can also be added. Stir well, take a mouthful, gargle and spit out. Stir again and repeat. It is important to stir the mixture before each mouthful so as to redisperse the oils. Gargling should be done twice a day for best results.

The procedure for mouthwashes is the same as for gargling, except that the liquid is swished around inside the mouth (rather than at the back of the throat) for 30 seconds before spitting out.

▷ **Adding a few drops of an antibacterial oil to a glass of water makes an effective gargle mix.**

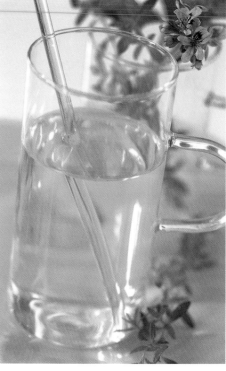

△ **When using a mouthwash, make sure the oils are well stirred in the water before each sip.**

safety
- For children and the elderly the essential oil quantities should be halved.

drinks

To use essential oils in drinks, the oils must be organic and mixed in a suitable carrier.

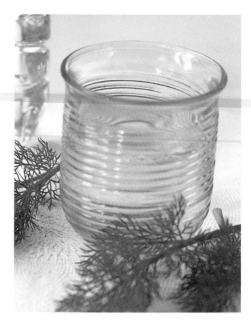

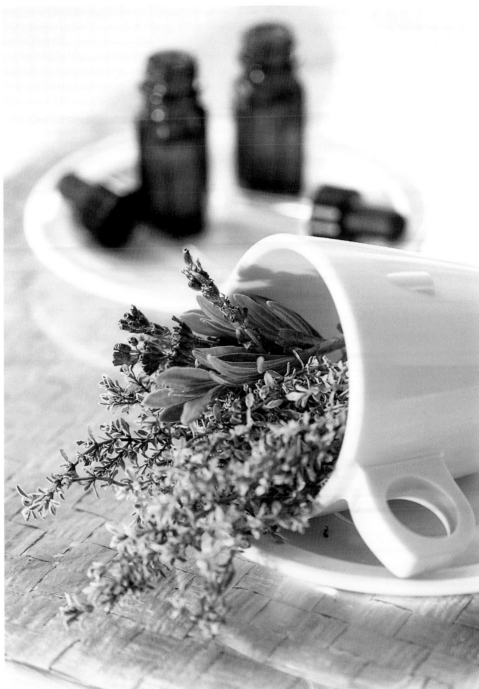

▷ Organic plants are grown without the use of chemicals. When taking oils internally, it is important to use only those of therapeutic and certified organic quality.

You are advised first to consult a qualified aromatologist or an aromatherapist working alongside a medical doctor. If you wish to use essential oils in water or tea at home without taking professional advice, it is imperative that the essential oils, and the dosage and time scales recommended in this book are strictly adhered to.

water

Drinking plenty of water is good for us. If you are not fond of water as a drink, put 2 drops of an essential oil such as lemon or orange into 1 litre (1¾ pints) of water in a bottle and shake well. For a healthy digestive system, use 1 drop each of peppermint and fennel oil and mix as before. Shake the bottle before drinking. In conjunction with healthy eating habits, 1 drop each of grapefruit and/or cypress, used as before, can help weight loss as part of a slimming and exercise programme.

teas

Only aromatologists are able to prescribe essential oils for internal, medicinal use. Tea is not a medicine, however, but a pleasant drink. If the tea tastes too strong when the oils are added, dilute it with more water.

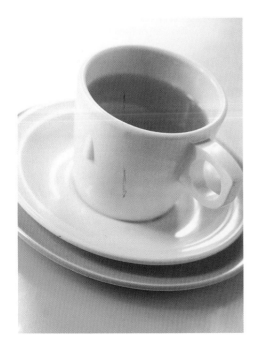

Tannin-free china tea or rooibos (red bush) tea make the best bases. Put 2–3 drops of essential oil on to the tea leaves or tea bag, add 1 litre (1¾ pints) of hot water, stir well, then remove the tea leaves or bag. The tea will taste better without milk. Never pour essential oil directly into tea: it will be too strong, and the oils will not disperse. Any tea not drunk immediately can be stored in the fridge and reheated as necessary.

For digestive disorders, a cup of tea drunk two or three times a day is a very gentle and effective remedy. Common

◁ Teas made with essential oils can be a pleasant way of enjoying the healing properties of plants.

urinary tract problems, such as cystitis, respond well, as do insomnia and pain from arthritic joints.

safety

- Use only organic essential oils of therapeutic quality for adding to drinks.
- Absolutes or resins should never be ingested.
- These methods should not be used on children, but are suitable for the elderly.
- Never put essential oils directly into a cup of tea or glass of water. Otherwise, the drink will taste far too strong and will be very unpleasant. The oils should be used only by the methods stated.

Aromatherapy massage techniques

Touch is the most basic human impulse, and massage is a therapeutic extension of touch dating back to ancient times. Hippocrates said that "rubbing loosens a joint that is too rigid", and when we hurt ourselves, our first reaction is to rub the pain away.

To experience a massage under qualified and caring hands is a relaxing experience in itself and it can only be enhanced by the addition of essential oils. If you cannot have treatment by a professional aromatherapist, there are some simple massage techniques you can practise at home on yourself or on a partner, using essential oils for beneficial results. Three simple self-massage techniques follow, together with a routine for Swiss Reflex Therapy (SRT) and useful tips for blending essential oils at home.

Neck and shoulder treatment

Day-to-day stresses and anxieties often manifest themselves as tension in the neck and shoulder muscles, and treating this area can bring immediate benefits. One of the best times to work on your neck and shoulders is just before going to bed, especially if stress or insomnia are a problem. This will help to relax you before going to sleep and will put your body into a healing mode. Prepare your choice of essential oils with a carrier lotion or oil (*see* Preparing Oils). Wear loose clothing or a towel, and remove all jewellery for comfort. Apply a little of the oil mix to both shoulders and begin the massage.

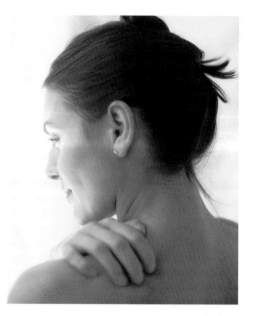

◁ **2** Keeping your hand in this position (palm on collarbone and fingers on shoulder muscle), feel with your fingers for any hard tension spots along the muscle and apply firm circular pressure to these with the pads of your three middle fingers. Be careful not to exceed an acceptable pain threshold.

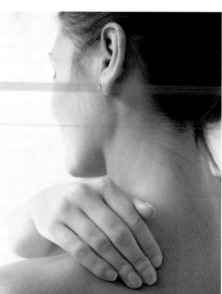

◁ **3** Take your fingers up your neck, repeating the circular movements with your three fingers where there are painful nodules. Repeat steps 2 and 3 if the area is still painful, and finish with several firm circles, as in step 1. Repeat the massage on the opposite shoulder, using your other hand.

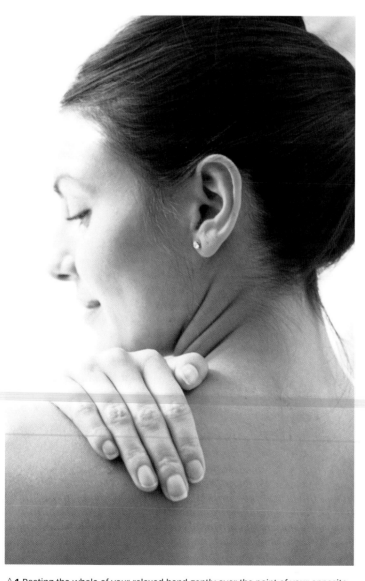

△**1** Resting the whole of your relaxed hand gently over the point of your opposite shoulder, move your hand firmly along the top of the shoulder until you reach the neck, then return to the shoulder point. Repeat this circle several times.

Headache treatment

It is instinctive to rub your temples or forehead when you have a headache. Giving yourself a head massage with one or more appropriate essential oils in a carrier lotion or oil can make the massage more effective.

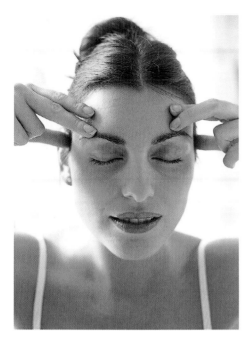

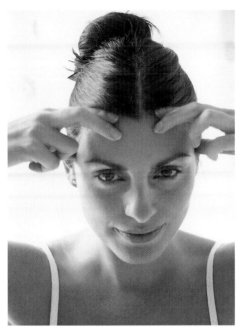

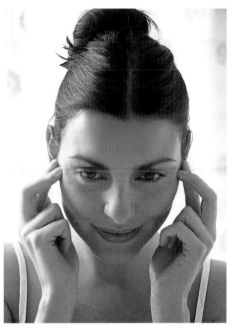

△ **1** Dab a little of the essential oil mix on your fingertips and place your fingers and thumbs at the temples. Place the length of your fingers on to your forehead and move them firmly from the centre towards the temples, returning back to the centre. Repeat several times.

△ **2** Keeping your thumbs in the same position, make circular movements from the centre of the top of your forehead to the upper temple, using only the cushions of your three middle fingers.

△ **3** Repeat these circles 1 cm (½ in) lower down the forehead, again moving from the centre to the temples. Repeat the circles, doing the last one at eyebrow level. With thumbs positioned as before, "glue" your fingers in the temple hollows and make firm circles which move the skin of the temples over the bone beneath. Repeat step 1.

Scalp treatment

A scalp massage is not only very relaxing, but is also very helpful for anyone who is worried about thinning hair, as it stimulates the hair roots. The roots can become starved of nourishment when the scalp muscle becomes too tight – such as through stress, for example – causing the hair to become thin and weak.

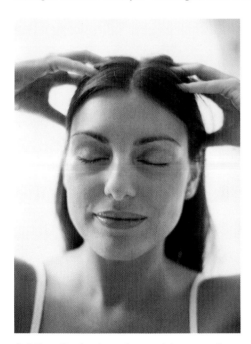

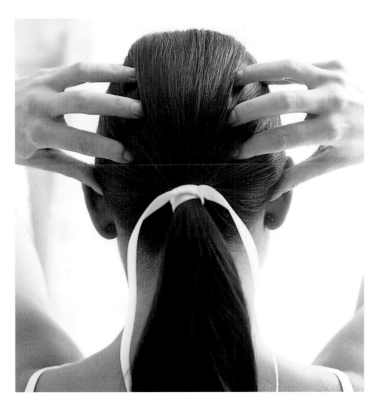

◁ **2** Place the hands on another part of the scalp and repeat. Carry on until the whole scalp has been covered. Repeat steps 1 and 2 several times.

△ **1** Place the thumbs at the top of the ears and "glue" the fingers to the scalp, moving it firmly and slowly over the bone beneath.

Swiss reflex therapy (SRT)

Historical evidence suggests that treatment involving the foot reflexes is as ancient as massage. Reflexology uses the energy flow lines in the body which culminate as reflex points in the feet, hands, ears and tongue. Each reflex point represents a particular organ or part of the body. If any malfunction occurs in the body, a blockage will occur in the energy pathway, and tiny crystalline deposits are formed at the reflex point representing the malfunctioning area. A reflexologist can feel these blockages and reflexology treatment aims to break them down. If you have acute or recurrent health problems, you are advised to consult a qualified reflexologist: the treatment is not only relaxing, but it can bring effective, lasting relief from symptoms.

Foot reflexes can be used as an aid to health by using Swiss Reflex Therapy. SRT is not reflexology, although it does manipulate the foot reflexes, which are massaged in a particular way. The therapy was devised by the author in Switzerland in 1987. It enables people with bronchial or spinal problems to treat themselves at home.

Ideally, attending a practical SRT course is the best way to learn, although the basic principles are more simple to learn than reflexology. SRT can be used at home for self-treatment and, with daily practice, positive results are achieved fairly quickly.

Use a bland moisturizing cream base and add essential oils: 30 drops of essential oil to every 30 ml (2 tbsp) of the cream. Vegetable oil is not suitable for use in SRT.

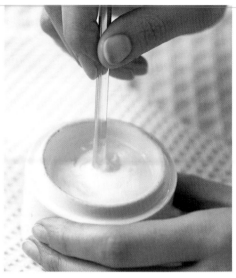

△ Swiss Reflex Treatment takes an equal number of drops of essential oil to millilitres of base cream. Stir the cream well after adding your chosen oil.

REFLEXOLOGY CHART

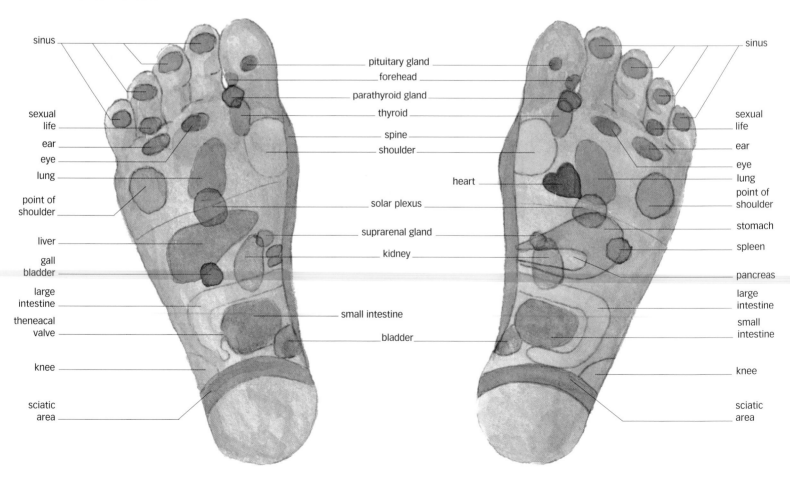

RIGHT FOOT   LEFT FOOT

Swiss reflex therapy

Always begin a treatment with the solar plexus reflex area, to relax the body, and end with the kidney–bladder area to help eliminate any released toxins.

The first time you experience pressure on a blocked reflex, the pain may be quite severe and is usually made worse by any stress you are under at the time. You should work only to your own pain threshold and massage the problematic reflex for one full minute, when you will find that the pain diminishes and gradually disappears altogether. If there is no pain, you are either not on the right reflex, not pressing hard enough, or there is no problem with the part of the body which that reflex represents.

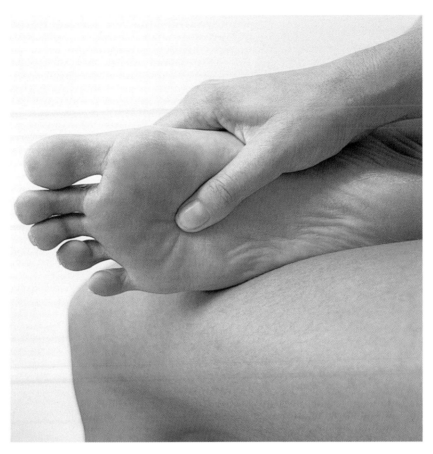

◁ **1** Rest your right foot on the knee of your left leg and massage the solar plexus reflex area with the whole length of your right thumb in a circular motion. Work as firmly as your pain tolerance level will allow, and hold on to the toes with your left hand if you find it easier. Keep circling, maintaining the same pressure until you feel it easing. Continue until the discomfort has completely gone. If it still feels painful after one minute, the original pressure may have been too strong.

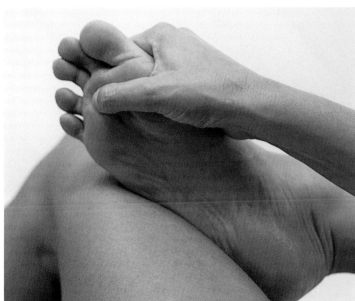

△ **2** Using circular movements again, massage any reflex areas which present a problem: for example, the lung area if you have bronchial problems, the digestive system for constipation (massaging in a clockwise direction), and the spinal areas for backache, muscular pains, rheumatism or arthritis. For a long area like the spine, do a small area at a time, moving down and repeating until all the spine has been covered. Change your hand position depending on the reflex being treated.

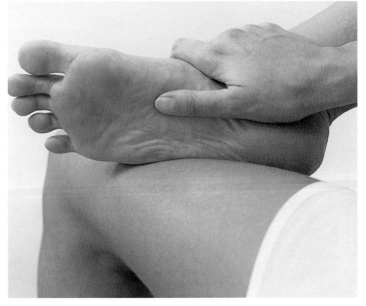

△ **3** When you have covered the relevant problem areas, massage with the full length of your right thumb in a firm oval movement. Again, hold the toes with your left hand if you find it easier. Follow the kidney-urethra-bladder: the pressure should be from kidney to bladder, with no pressure being applied on the return half of the circle. Repeat the whole three-step sequence on your left foot, changing your hands over for easier movement.

Preparing oils for application

Essential oils can be added to a range of carrier bases: vegetable oils, unscented lotion or cream. The choice of base depends on how the mixture is to be used, and is also a matter of personal preference.

types of carrier oil

There are many suitable vegetable oils, each with its own benefit. Unrefined, cold-pressed oils are the best for aromatherapy. The basic oils are widely available, while special and macerated oils are available from suppliers. As a guide, use 15–20 drops of essential oil in 50 ml of the base oil for mixtures to be applied to the skin. Reduce the ratio to 1:10 for preparations to be used on the face.

basic oils

Sunflower *Helianthus annuus*

This oil is taken from the seeds of the giant yellow sunflower. It can relieve eczema and dermatitis, lower blood cholesterol, soothe rheumatism, and ease leg ulcers, sprains and bruises. It may also have diuretic properties.

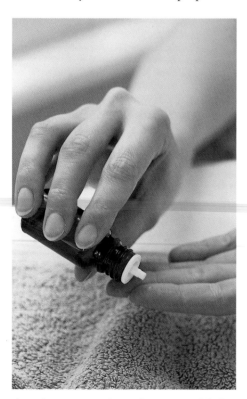

△ **Apply one or two drops of neat essential oil direct to the skin to soothe cuts, bites and stings.**

Sweet almond *Prunus amygdalis* var. *dulcis*

Almond oil is taken from the kernel of the almond nut, but it is difficult to obtain cold-pressed almond oil. This oil alleviates inflamed and irritated skin, helps to relieve constipation, lowers blood cholesterol, and is good for eczema, psoriasis and dry skin.

special oils

These can all be used alone or as 25 per cent of a basic carrier oil.

Evening primrose *Oenethera biennis*

Yellow evening primrose flowers open at dusk, one circle of flowers at a time. The flowers open so quickly that the buds can be watched as they open. The flowers' seeds are cold-pressed when the stem has finished flowering. Evening primrose oil will relieve arthritis, lower blood cholesterol, help PMS, and soothe wounds. It is excellent for eczema, psoriasis and dry skin, and is said to have a beneficial effect on wrinkles.

Hazelnut *Corylus avellana*

Cold-pressed hazelnuts yield an amber coloured oil. Hazelnut oil has astringent properties and can be used to relieve acne, stimulate circulation and protect against the harmful effects of the sun.

Jojoba *Simmondsia chinensis*

Jojoba is not an oil but a liquid wax, which gives it excellent keeping qualities. Jojoba is an analgesic with anti-inflammatory properties, and it will soothe arthritis and rheumatism, acne, eczema, psoriasis, dry skin and sunburn. Jojoba is good for the scalp, and is a useful addition to shampoo.

Rose hip *Rosa canina*

These small berries produce a syrup, a rich source of Vitamin C, and a golden-red oil. Rose hip oil is anti-aging and will help to regenerate tissue. It softens mature skin, and is good to use for burns, scars and eczema.

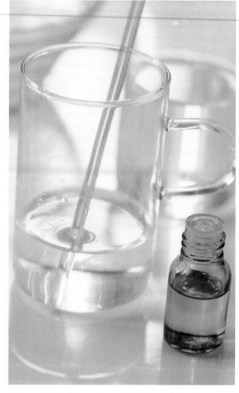

△ **Essential oils can be added to cold spring water to make your own customized skin toner. Choose the right oils for your skin type.**

macerated oils

The process of macerating (soaking) plants in olive or sunflower oil enhances base oils with the plants' therapeutic properties. These macerated carrier oils can be added to a base vegetable oil, lotion or cream to enrich it. Macerated melissa and lime oils can also be used to enrich base oils.

Calendula *Calendula officinalis*

Often referred to as marigold (although it is not related to French marigold, *Tagetes minuta*), Calendula has anti-inflammatory and astringent properties, and can relieve broken and varicose veins. Apply directly in undiluted form to ease sprains and bruises.

St John's wort *Hypericum perforatum*

With its analgesic and anti-inflammatory properties, St John's wort will help to relieve haemorrhoids, sprains, bruises and arthritis, and can heal burns, sunburn and wounds.

carrier lotion and cream

Unperfumed lotion, which is made from emulsified oil and water, can be used instead of vegetable oil as a carrier base. Lotion is particularly good for all self-application techniques as it is non-greasy. Use a cream if a base richer than a lotion is needed.

To prepare a blend for use on the body, mix 15–20 drops of essential oil with 50 ml (2 fl oz) of lotion or cream. For a blend to be used on the face, mix 5 drops of essential oil per 50 ml (2 fl oz) lotion or cream. For a foot reflex treatment (*see* Swiss Reflex Therapy) add 50 drops of oil to 50 ml (2 fl oz) of cream.

safety note

Except for a cream blend to be used in Swiss Reflex Therapy, use only half the specified quantity of essential oils in any base carrier – vegetable oil, lotion or cream – if the mixture is to be used on children and the elderly.

Preparing a blend for the body using vegetable oil

Vegetable oils are excellent carriers for massage. The essential oils readily dissolve in them, and they allow the hands to move continuously on the skin without dragging or slipping. Mineral oil, such as baby oil, is from a mineral, not a vegetable source. It aims to protects the skin by keeping moisture out and will not allow essential oils to penetrate: it is not suitable as a base oil.

ingredients
- essential oils
- vegetable carrier oil

equipment
- screw-top bottle
- label and marker pen

tips

Care should be taken not to use too much of the mixed oil as it can stain sheets and clothes. To stop too much oil coming out at a time, place your fingers over the top of the bottle, tipping it against them. Apply the fingers to the area to be treated, repeating only if you need more oil.

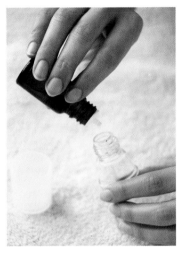

△ **1** Pour 15–20 drops of your chosen essential oil or oils into a 50 ml (2 fl oz) screw-top bottle.

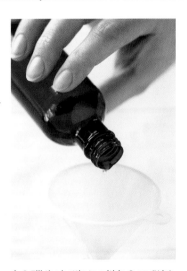

△ **2** Fill the bottle to within 2 cm (¾ in) of the top with your chosen vegetable carrier oil. Use a funnel, if preferred, to avoid any unnecessary spillage

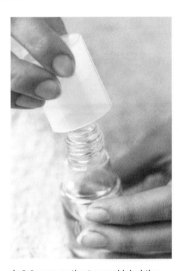

△ **3** Screw on the top and label the bottle with the quantity of each oil used, what the mixture is to be used for, your name and the date.

Preparing a blend for the body using lotion

A bland, non-greasy lotion is preferable to oil as it is less messy and is absorbed quickly by the skin. A lotion base is better for self-application techniques, as a vegetable oil bottle will become greasy and can easily slip through your fingers.

ingredients
- bland white lotion
- vegetable oil (optional)
- essential oils

equipment
- screw-top jar or bottle
- label and marker pen

tips

Prepare a blend with a cream base in the same way. For a preparation to use on the face, mix 50 ml (2 fl oz) of the base lotion or cream with only 5 drops of your chosen essential oil.

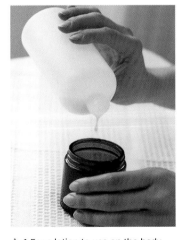

△ **1** For a lotion to use on the body, fill a 50 ml (2 fl oz) jar or bottle three-quarters full with an unperfumed white lotion, or a lotion mixed with a little vegetable oil, if preferred.

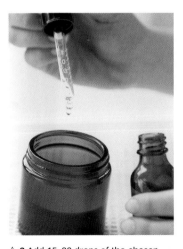

△ **2** Add 15–20 drops of the chosen essential oil or oil blend. Screw on the top and shake thoroughly. Add the rest of the lotion but do not fill right to the top, to allow room for reshaking.

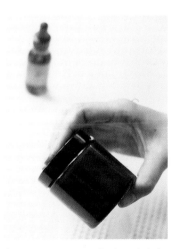

△ **3** Screw the top on firmly and shake again. Label with the contents, use, your name and the date. For a facial lotion, mix 50 ml (2 fl oz) of the base lotion with 5 drops of essential oil.

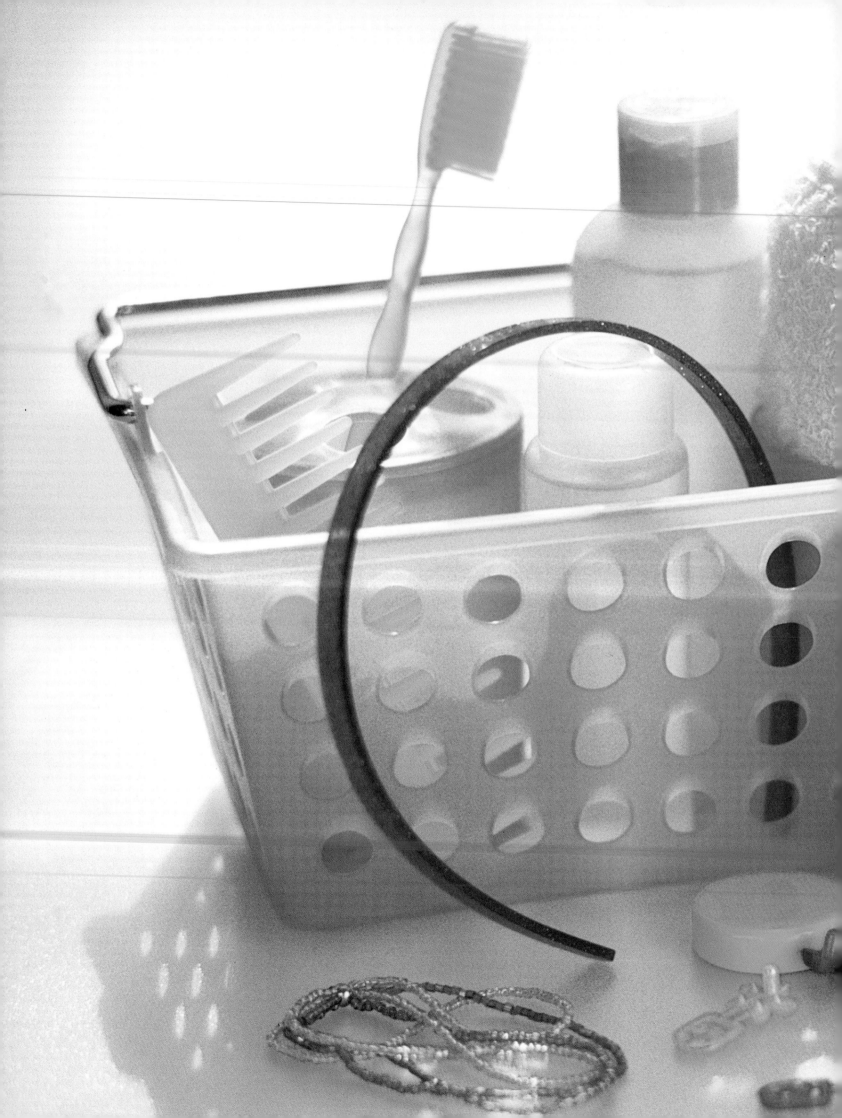

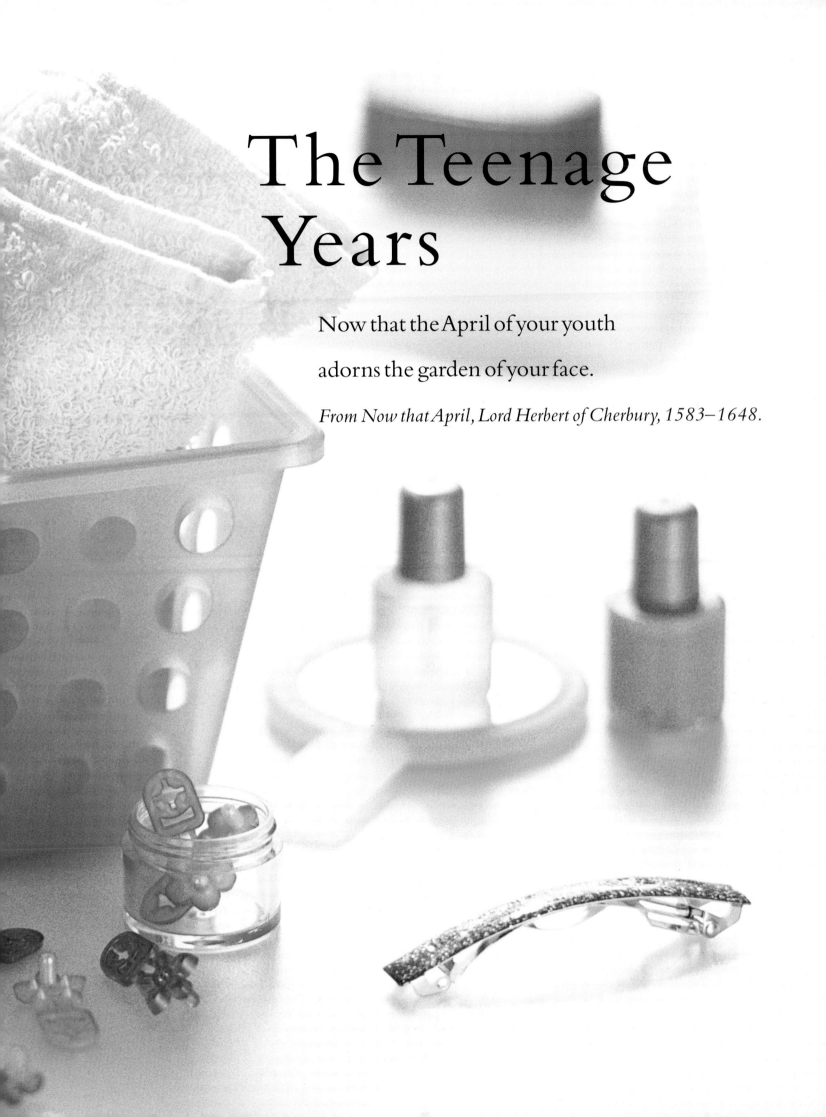

The Teenage Years

Now that the April of your youth

adorns the garden of your face.

From Now that April, Lord Herbert of Cherbury, 1583–1648.

Aromatherapy in adolescence

The actual rate at which children grow up varies greatly and there can be several years difference in the age at which individual children reach puberty. With the advent of puberty, both health and emotional patterns begin to change. The pituitary gland, responsible for the body's physical growth, begins to release hormones which stimulate the ovaries or testicles to produce eggs or sperm. As soon as these hormonal changes begin to take place, the girl starts to become a young woman and the boy a young man.

For a girl, one of the more obvious signs of becoming a young woman is marked by her developing breasts and by the onset of her periods. This can be a difficult time as she either adjusts to the physical changes that are taking place, or worries because they are happening too fast or not fast

ESSENTIAL OILS AND THE SKIN

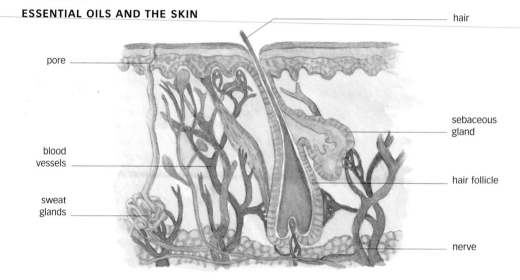

pore

blood vessels

sweat glands

hair

sebaceous gland

hair follicle

nerve

△ **A basic understanding of how the skin operates will help you to take care of it.**

enough. Essential oils can be extremely useful to alleviate some of the physical discomforts and emotional aspects often associated with puberty and menstruation (*see* The Reproductive Years).

▷ **Being a teenager is not always easy. Hormone imbalances can lead to extreme mood swings and problems with both the hair and the skin.**

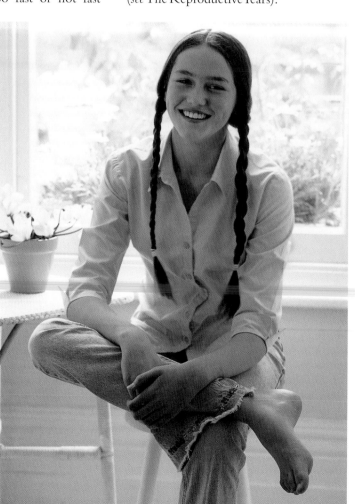

The teenage years are typically turbulent times. A girl's body is rapidly growing and changing in new and startling ways, and her hormones are likely to be affecting both her body and her mood. Hormonal changes trigger an imbalance of sebum in the skin (usually increasing the amount produced), which can lead to greasy skin and hair. This can be awkward at a time when a young woman is becoming aware of her appearance, and of the effect she has on the opposite sex, and feelings of inadequacy are common. The associated emotions of anxiety, resentment, fear and jealousy can all increase stress levels and trigger further reactions in the hair, skin and/or nails.

Essential oils can be very useful both in alleviating unsettled emotional states and treating the skin and hair problems themselves. Aromatherapy, used correctly, forms just one part of a holistic approach to health, and this approach should take into account the girl's nutrition and lifestyle habits, as well as any stressful or worrying external circumstances or events in her life, before the essential oils can be chosen. Now that she is no longer a child, a teenager needs to feel in control of her life, and looking after her health is a good way to begin.

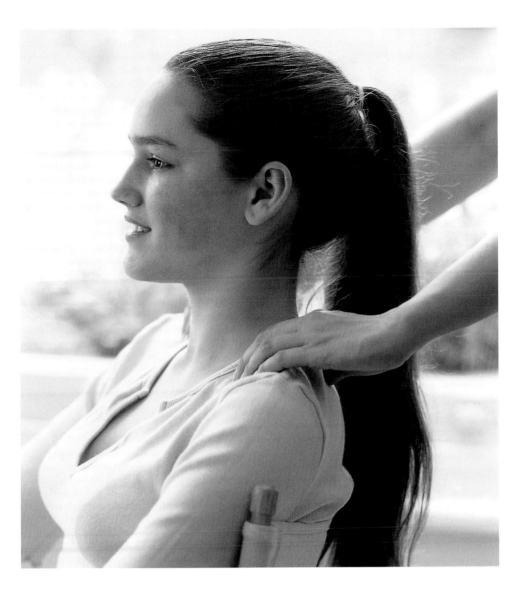

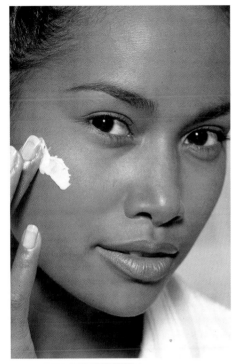

◁ Receiving a shoulder masage is a pleasant and effective way of relieving stress and tension in the neck and shoulders. Ask a friend to gently rub and knead any knotty or tight areas.

△ Experiment with adding oils to your own skin creams and see which combinations work best.

stress and anxiety

Apart from the changes taking place within her own body, life in the outside world can also be problematic for today's teenager. External circumstances, which are beyond her control, can be difficult to manage. If a parent changes job, for example, the family may have to move house and area. This means a new school, with a new teacher, and no immediate friends – all at a time when the academic workload is increasing and exams are becoming a reality. School may also be stressful because of bullying. This affects many teenagers, who exist in a perpetual state of fear and feel they are unable to talk to anyone about it.

There may also be problems within the family: heavy arguments between parents, between the teenager and her parents, or between siblings. For example, teenagers may feel rivalry or jealousy towards a brother or sister who seems to be given more of a parent's love and attention, and receives special treats and favours.

In many societies, the divorce rate is increasing and many modern-day children are "shared" between parents. It is debatable whether it is more stressful to the child to live with parents who don't get on and who argue, or to be caught between two homes.

Growing up involves finding out who you are and having your own ideas and opinions. Problems can arise when parents and their teenage daughter don't see eye-to-eye, and angry fights at home become a routine part of life. Teenagers face strong peer pressure to conform to current trends. This usually involves wearing the "right" clothes, and going to the "right" places for entertainment and holidays. All of these things cost money and can cause tension within the family.

Whatever the reason for stress or anxiety, however, there are numerous relaxing or sedative essential oils which can help (*see* Coping with Stress). These are best used in the bath or, for more immediate results, by inhalation (*see* Aromatherapy Techniques).

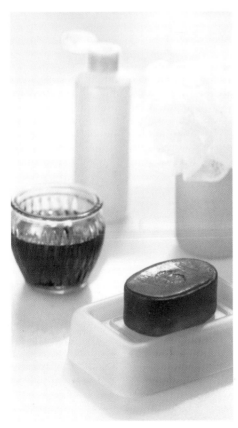

△ Now is a good time to start a daily beauty regime and have fun taking care of yourself.

Everyday skincare

Embarrassing and unsightly skin conditions can be improved by following a healthy diet and a regular skin-cleansing routine using suitable products. The important thing is to follow both of these recommendations if you want to see positive, lasting results.

lifestyle changes

A good starting point is to make a record of your dietary intake each day for a week. By studying this, you will be able to make any necessary adjustments. Try substituting fresh fruit for crisps and chocolate, or fresh juices and/or mineral water for carbonated, sugary drinks. At the same time, monitor improvements to your skin.

If you support yourself by taking aromatherapy baths to relieve stress and follow the skin-cleansing regime below, you should see visible results within a week. If you do not, it may be because the diet and/or care treatments have not been strictly followed.

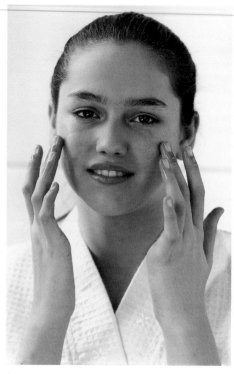

△ **Regularly cleansing and moisturizing your face will keep your complexion at its best**.

Remember, too, that acne is often worse just before menstruation, and that teenage acne usually subsides by the early twenties.

problem skin

The hormonal changes of puberty lead to increased production of sebum by the sebaceous glands in the skin. From the normal, peach-like skin of childhood, a young woman may find her skin (particularly on her face) changing in texture. The pores become enlarged and more open and the skin becomes oily – particularly on the forehead and in a "T-panel" leading down the nose and on to the chin. These open pores are a breeding ground for bacteria, leading to spots, pimples and blackheads, which is why a regular and effective skin-cleansing routine becomes so important.

A spotty skin can become a problem if it develops into acne (*Acne vulgaris*). This is a medical condition and requires special care.

Daily skincare routine

To see an immediate improvement to the skin, a five minute skincare routine should be established and carried out twice a day. Essential oils added to unperfumed creams or lotions can be useful for treating difficult skin conditions and to help with the added emotional difficulties of low self-confidence. With perseverance (and improved lifestyle habits), this routine has proved to be extremely effective. Once the skin begins to improve, stress is reduced and a positive, rather than a negative, cycle is created.

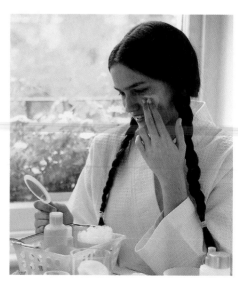

△ **1** Cleanse the skin with a light, water-soluble cleansing milk. Make your own by blending 1 drop each of rosemary, lavender and geranium oils into 30 ml (2 tbsp) base lotion. Rinse off with cold water.

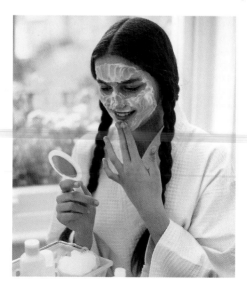

△ **2** Make a gentle, purifying mask by adding 2 drops each of cedarwood, juniper and lemon essential oils to 30 ml (2 tbsp) base cream. Apply to face and leave for ten minutes. Rinse off thoroughly with cold water.

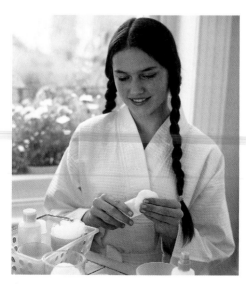

△ **3** Add 3 drops each of lemon and geranium oils to 50 ml (2 fl oz) distilled water. Wipe over the face and neck as a tonic. Follow with a moisturizing lotion mixed with 2 drops of hazelnut oil.

▷ The feet are prone to patches of dry, rough skin. Moisturizing your feet on a regular basis will help to keep them smooth and soft.

▽ Drinking plenty of mineral water can vastly improve your overall health and vitality.

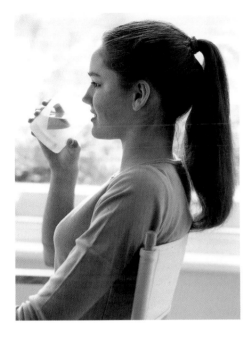

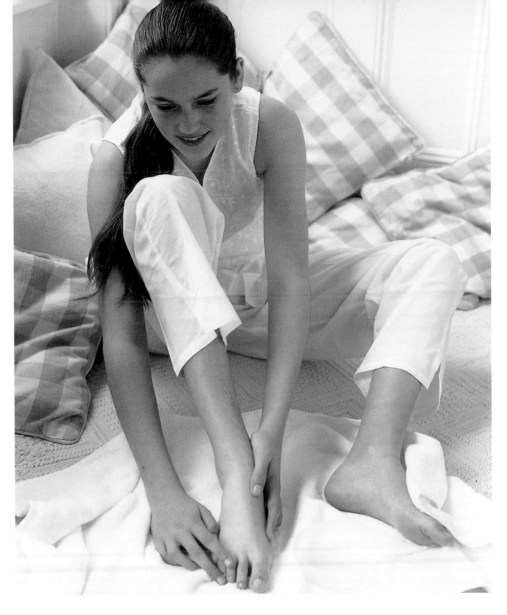

teenage acne

Acne is caused when excessive amounts of sebum form a blockage at the skin's surface on the face, shoulders and back. Cysts, blackheads and red pustules develop, which can lead to pockmark scars. It is difficult to improve the skin once these scars appear.

The rise in the incidence and severity of teenage acne seems to be connected with some aspects of today's modern culture.

Insufficient fresh fruit and vegetables in the diet, chemical additives in food, and air pollution all cause a toxin overload which puts extra strain on the body. Taking good care of your skin and body will really help.

tips for healthy skin
• Stick to a suitable daily skincare routine.
• Exercise for half an hour three times a week.
• Eat lots of fresh fruit and vegetables.
• Drink 6–8 glasses of mineral water a day.

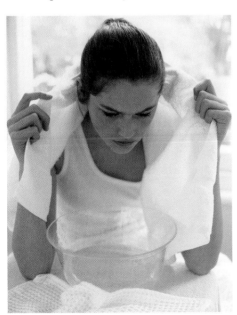

△ Regular steam inhalations with juniper can help clear blocked pores or blackheads.

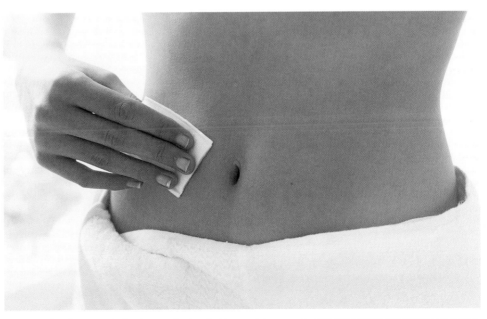

△ Stomach ache or period pains can be treated by applying a compress using basil, lavender and sweet marjoram. A piece of soft cotton or linen soaked in a water-oil mix makes a good compress.

Caring for hair and nails

Both the hair and nails are made of keratin, a modified skin tissue, and both are present to protect us from harm. The hair and nails benefit from good nutrition, and care with essential oils can improve their appearance.

teenage hair

Hair problems for teenagers will often mean greasy hair. Greasy hair needs frequent washing with a suitable shampoo to prevent the excess oil from causing spots around the hairline. However, the rubbing action on the scalp stimulates the sebaceous glands to produce more sebum and can make the problem worse. If you have greasy hair, shampoo it no more than once a day. Add an astringent essential oil to an unperfumed shampoo for your own aromatherapy treatment at home. Take care to apply the shampoo to the hair and not the scalp.

▷ **If your hair lacks lustre, try adding the appropriate oils to an unperfumed conditioner base. After shampooing, gently comb the mix through to the ends of your hair.**

Hair loss can also be a problem for some young women. This can be brought on by the stress of exams and personal worries, and also by harsh treatment of hair that is already weak, such as dragging it back too tightly from the forehead with hairbands. Mixing essential oils with your shampoo can help to strengthen weak hair. Handle hair with care, and ease it forward slightly before adding hairbands and accessories.

conditioning

The condition of our hair is crucial to how we look, and good hair treatment brings its own rewards. Hair should be trimmed regularly – with no more than 1 cm (½ in) removed – to keep the ends strong. This is especially important with long hair: the more often long hair is trimmed, the faster it will grow and the better it will look.

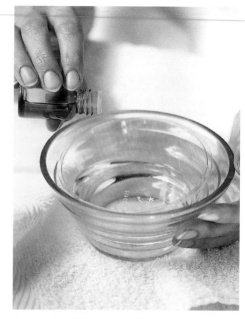

△ **Lavender oil is very useful for treating difficult nail conditions. Add a 2–3 drops to 5 ml (1 tsp) carrier oil and use as required.**

If your hair is in poor condition, use a separate conditioner: products which aim to combine a shampoo with a conditioner are rarely effective as they cannot do both jobs well. Add the essential oils your hair needs to an unperfumed, basic conditioner. Apply the mixture to your hair and scalp after shampooing and towel-drying. Cover with a plastic bag to keep in the heat, and leave for 30 minutes before rinsing well.

tips for healthy hair

- Add 8–10 drops of essential oils to 50 ml (2 fl oz) of unfragranced shampoo (not baby shampoo – it is not especially mild).
- Give yourself a daily scalp massage with soothing essential oils to arrest and prevent early hair loss.

nailcare

Nail-biting is often connected to stress and has a strong emotional component. It can be a difficult habit to break. Because teenage girls are often concerned with appearance, the desire for beautiful, manicured nails may help to overcome the problem.

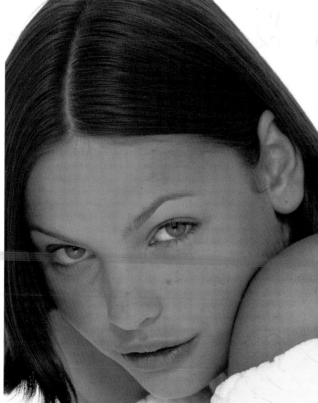

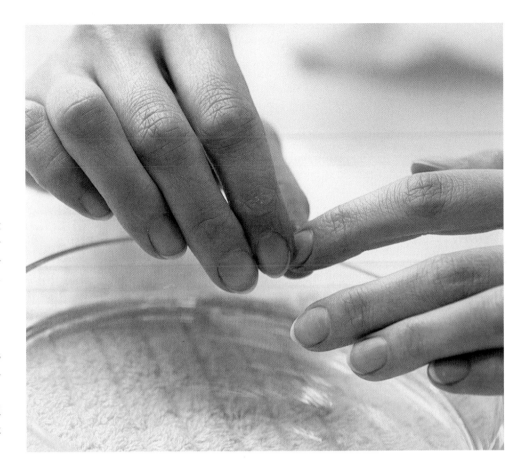

▷ Strong and beautiful nails begin at the cuticle. Use an oil mix and gently massage it on to the cuticle and surrounding area daily. After three months, you will see improvement in your nails.

To encourage strong, healthy nails, you have to care for the cuticle as well as the nail, as this is where nail growth begins. Health disorders can cause ridging and thinning of the nails. Psoriasis and fungus under the nail tips can be treated with lavender or geranium oils. As with skin and hair, the nails give an indication of inner health.

tips for healthy nails

- Discourage nail-biting by coating the nails daily with neat lavender oil. The unpleasant taste of the oil will stop the chewing.
- Apply neat lavender oil daily to the nail cuticle to improve the condition of weak nails. Results will show in three months.

Useful essential oils

essential oil	treatment
hair	
Caraway *Carum carvi*	stimulant, encourages hair growth, aids scalp problems.
Cedarwood *Cedrus atlantica*	antiseptic and stimulant to scalp, reduces greasy dandruff, helps to renew hair growth
Clary sage *Salvia sclarea*	regenerative, improves poor hair growth
Juniper *Juniperus communis*	antiseborrhoeic (greasy dandruff), antiseptic (greasy scalp)
Lemon *Citrus limon*	antibacterial, astringent (reduces greasy dandruff)
Rosemary *Rosmarinus officinalis*	stimulating to circulation, helps renew hair growth
Ylang ylang *Cananga odorata*	tonic to scalp, aids hair growth
nails	
Geranium *Pelargonium graveolens*	antifungal (athlete's foot, skin and nail fungi)
Lavender *Lavandula angustifolia*	antifungal (athlete's foot, skin and nail fungi), healing (strengthens weak nails)
Tea tree *Melaleuca alternifolia*	anti-infectious, antifungal (skin and nail infections)

essential oil	treatment
skin	
Geranium *Pelargonium graveolens*	cicatrizant (healing), useful for open acne
Juniper *Juniperus communis*	antiseborrhoeic, antiseptic
Lavender *Lavandula angustifolia*	antiseptic, cicatrizant (healing)
Lemon *Citrus limon*	antibacterial, astringent
Petitgrain *Citrus aurantium* var. *amara* (fol)	anti-inflammatory, antiseptic, useful for infected acne
Cedarwood *Cedrus atlantica*	antiseptic, cicatrizant, stimulant (skin and scalp problems)
stress	
Clary sage *Salvia sclarea*	calming
Geranium *Pelargonium graveolens*	relaxant (agitation, anxiety)
Lavender *Lavandula angustifolia*	calming and sedative
Lemon *Citrus limon*	calming and sedative
Petitgrain *Citrus aurantium* var. *amara* (fol)	balancing and calming
emotions	
Bergamot *Citrus bergamia*	sedative, neurotonic, cicatrizant, antispasmodic (anxiety, agitation, grief, fear, mood swings)

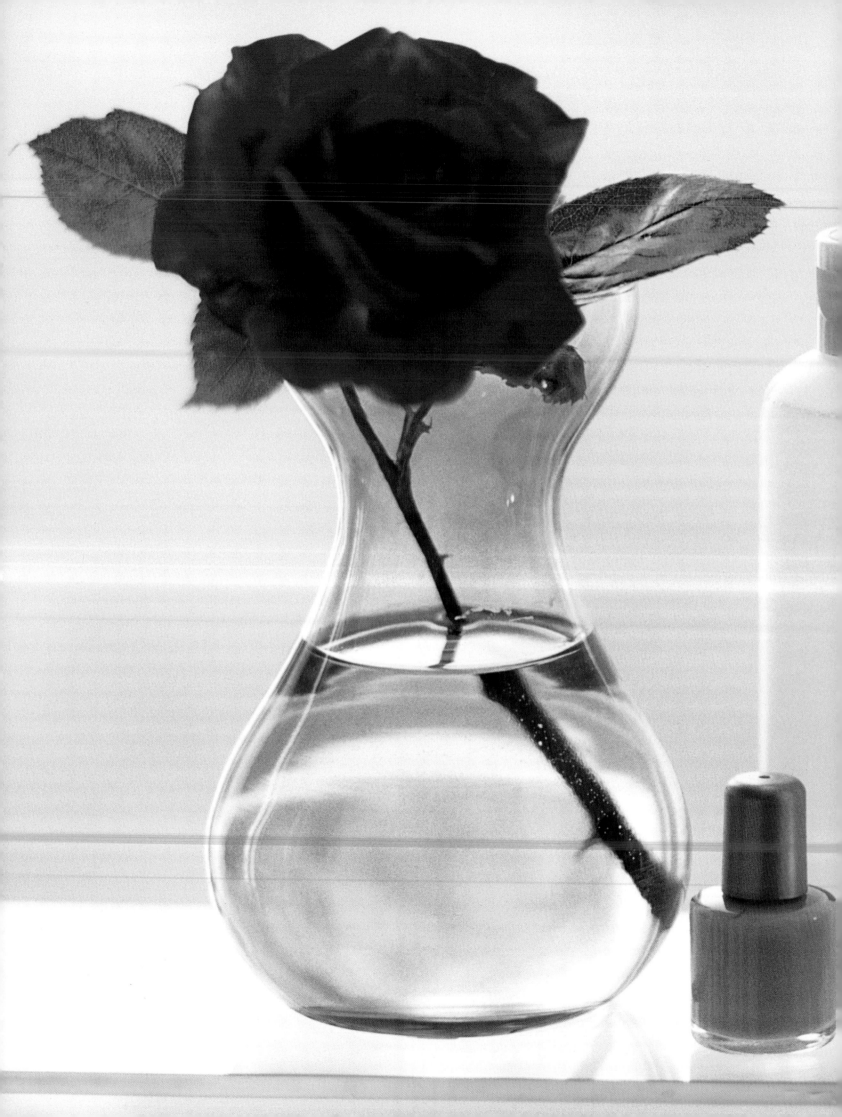

Beauty and Well-being

Here first she bathes, and round her body pours

Soft oils of fragrance and ambrosial showers.

From The Iliad, Homer, 8BC.

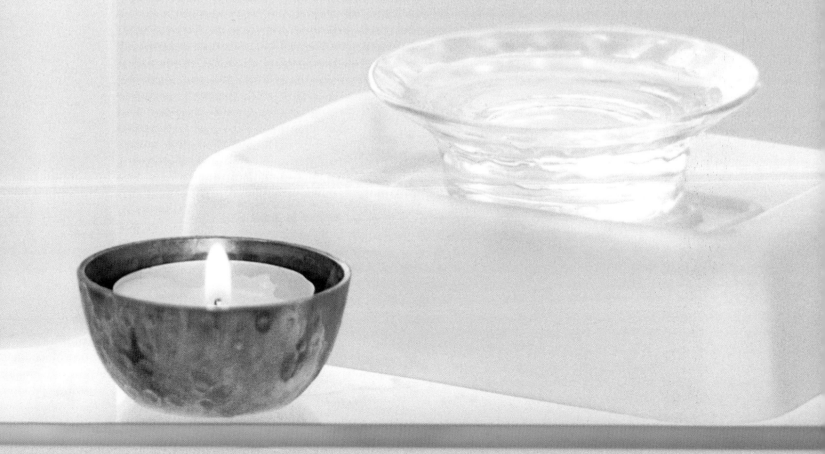

Looking after yourself

Looking and feeling good is important for most women. Commercial products can do much to treat beauty emergencies, but the only effective, long-term solution is optimum health in body and mind.

beautiful skin

A good complexion is a huge beauty asset: it helps a woman to look good and this, in turn, will boost morale. The skin is the largest organ of the body. It is always on display to the outside world and is worth taking care of. The skin has a slightly acid mantle, which keeps out harmful bacteria, and it is not a good idea to use excessively alkaline cleansers, such as soap, to wash the skin, as these destroy the necessary acid balance. The condition of the skin is a good indicator of general health within the body.

lifestyle

The condition of our skin is affected by our lifestyle and general well-being, including our diet, how much exercise we take, our work, our family and our mental attitude.

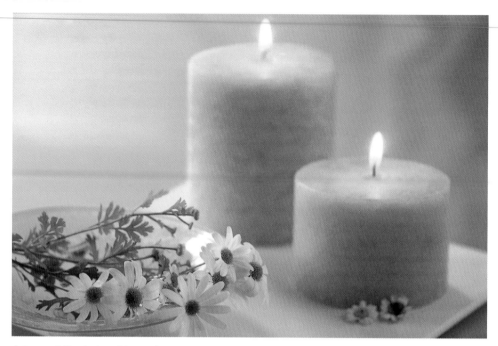

△ By carefully placing objects of natural beauty in your home, you can help your mind to relax and unwind. Soft candelight is traditionally associated with feelings of peace and harmony.

To some extent, we are what we eat. Our circulatory system carries the nutrients from our food around the body: without a healthy diet, the body's cells receive insufficient nutrition. Regular exercise is also important. A sedentary lifestyle, when combined with a lack of exercise, means that food nutrients are not transported around the body efficiently, and toxins in the lymphatic system are not completely eliminated. This can lead to cellulite and other problems in the body and with the skin. A diet which includes plenty of water, fresh fruit and vegetables will help to keep our bodies free from toxins and promote a blooming, clear complexion.

Our day-to-day environment can also affect our bodies. Most homes and offices are centrally heated, and this has a drying effect on skin and hair. Keeping a bowl of water beside each radiator will help to increase humidity. Women who spend a great deal of time outdoors should take care

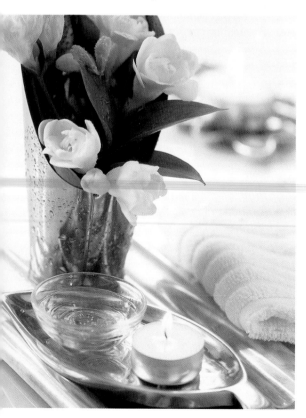

◁ Strategically placed oil and water mixes can increase humidity levels and also release aromas.

to protect their skin from excessive exposure to the sun, rain and wind: these are all damaging to the skin, and will promote wrinkles and early aging. Protect your skin from exposure to harmful ultraviolet rays, on the sunbed or outdoors, to reduce the risk of skin cancer.

Whether you are a working mother, a full-time mother, or a full-time career woman, feeling happy with what you do is important. This, in turn, is reflected in the condition of the skin, hair and nails. When we are unhappy, we tend to feel negative about ourselves and are more likely to focus on our tiny imperfections. This can leave us feeling even worse and creates a vicious cycle which can lead to depression. With a positive mental attitude, on the other hand, we feel happier and more buoyant, our stress levels decrease, and we look and feel in a healthier state.

the aging process

Like all other organs, the skin deteriorates with age. Typically this is characterized by the slowing down of cell regeneration, and

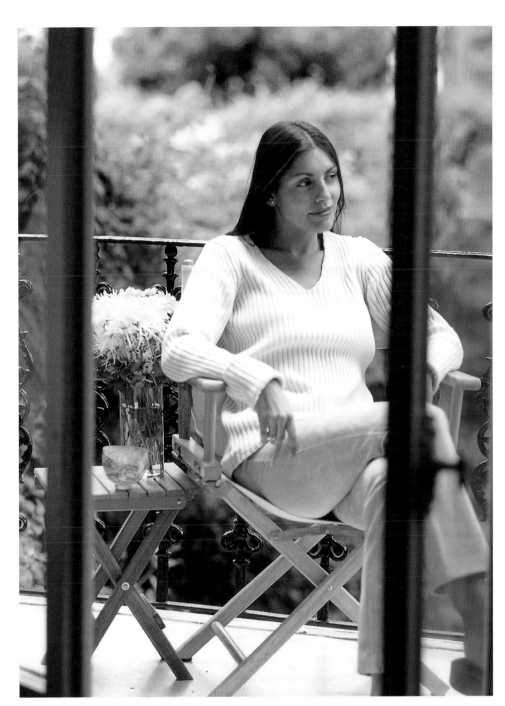

▷ Enjoying some quiet time alone each day
is important. It allows you to recharge your
batteries, giving you space for relaxation and
contemplation without any outside pressures.

the fact that dead skin cells gradually take longer to be discarded. As we grow older, our skin becomes less moist and loses its elasticity. Facial expressions are more likely to develop into wrinkle lines. As oestrogen production decreases during the menopause years (*see* The Menopause), there is a thinning and dehydration of the epidermis (the outer layer of the skin).

Many factors play a part in skin aging: heredity, menopause, occupation, exposure to the sun and wind, poor diet, alcohol-consumption, smoking, prolonged stress, insufficient sleep, even crash diets (which can cause wrinkles) and excessive washing (which can dehydrate the skin). The aging process is also partly due to the formation of free radicals in the body, developed from a reaction between sunlight and oxygen. These molecules are unstable and, in their search to stabilize, reactions occur in the body which can cause cellular destruction, resulting in skin aging and internal disease.

Aging is beyond our control, but we can help to minimize its effects by giving our bodies the best attention possible. Lifestyle factors need to be addressed and then supported by a daily care regime

with suitable lotions and creams, which can help to improve the elasticity and appearance of the skin, hair and nails. Protection can be taken against the negative effects of the weather and central heating.

It has been shown that essential oils can be used successfully to combat the effects of aging. Research studies have shown that many essential oils have cell regenerative properties, and essential oil products help to promote a much healthier, younger-looking skin. The essential oil molecules penetrate the skin and are able to work at the germinative layer, where the new cells are formed. These improved cells eventually reach the surface of the skin where the appearance is vastly improved.

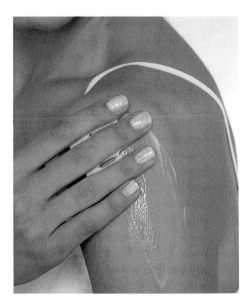

△ Apply a lotion containing analgesic essential oils to relieve aches and pains in the shoulders.

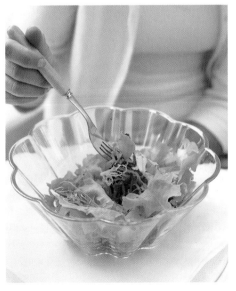

△ Eating plenty of fresh raw vegetables, fruits and salads will keep your energy levels high.

Daily skincare

The sooner a woman begins a good skincare routine, the more she will reap the benefits as she gets older. A good moisturizer is arguably the most important item in a woman's wardrobe – you can replace your clothes, but not your skin. It is well worth investing in an efficient, quality moisturizer that you like to use.

There is a vast array of commercial products available, designed for every skin permutation imaginable: teenage, normal, dry, oily, mature, sensitive, and allergy-prone skins. Although well-formulated cosmetics without essential oils may benefit the skin, a natural, quality range with added essential oils will increase the benefits.

choosing products

With aromatherapy, you should only have to choose between two basic product types because all essential oils are normalizing,

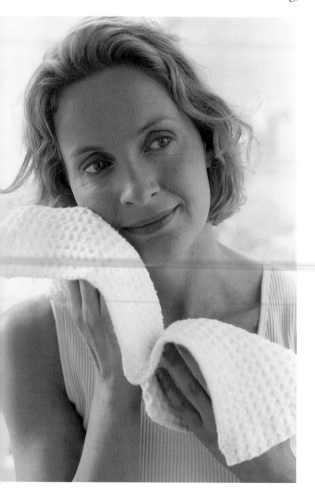

◁ **Always pat your face dry with a soft towel after rinsing. The skin on the face needs careful handling, whatever our age.**

giving exceptional care to the skin. If the skin is normal to oily, then look for a cleansing milk and moisturizing *lotion*. Choose cleansing and moisturizing *creams* when the skin is more dry and in need of nourishment. Look for products which have good quality bases and which don't contain alcohol, lanolin or other animal products. Night creams containing lanolin make your skin greasy, as the molecules are actually too big to penetrate the skin, and the cream will "sit" on top of your face all night, rubbing off on the pillow. Prepare your products with well chosen essential oils in a concentration of 0.5 per cent.

tips for healthy skin

If you wear make-up, it is important to cleanse your skin thoroughly before bed. In the morning, toner on cotton wool (cotton ball) is usually sufficient. Give yourself a treatment mask once a week. After a mask, you should moisturize twice, as masks draw out moisture as well as toxins. If you don't wear any make-up, a mask once a fortnight is usually sufficient.

If you don't wear make-up, use a mild toner only at night-time after cleansing. Moisturize first thing in the morning, after cleansing and toning.

creating your own products

To make your own skincare products, use unperfumed bases, adding the appropriate essential oils, 1 drop for each 10 ml (2 tsp) of carrier. Cold spring water is an excellent basic toner.

oily skin or acne

daytime base lotion with 10 per cent spring water added slowly while stirring.
night-time base lotion with 10 per cent hazelnut oil added slowly while stirring.

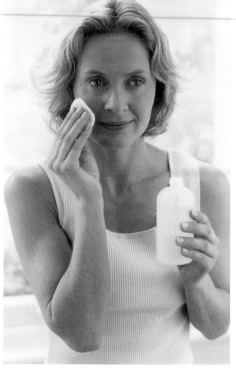

△ **Spring water can be used as a basic toner for all types of skin. Add your chosen essential oils.**

dry or mature skin

daytime base lotion with 25 per cent rose hip or jojoba oils added slowly while stirring.
night-time base cream with 50 per cent rose hip or jojoba, or the macerated oils of lime blossom or melissa added while stirring.

at the menopause

Try using hormone-like essential oils such as clary sage and niaouli which both have oestrogen-like properties.

skin disorders

A skin problem can arise from many causes, some of which may be more obvious than others. It may stem from an internal physical problem, such as poor digestion or painful periods, or from a mental problem, such as deep-rooted anxiety or grief. The effects of on-going mental and emotional stress can also cause skin problems, which in turn may aggravate the condition as we become worried, anxious and embarrassed about how others see us.

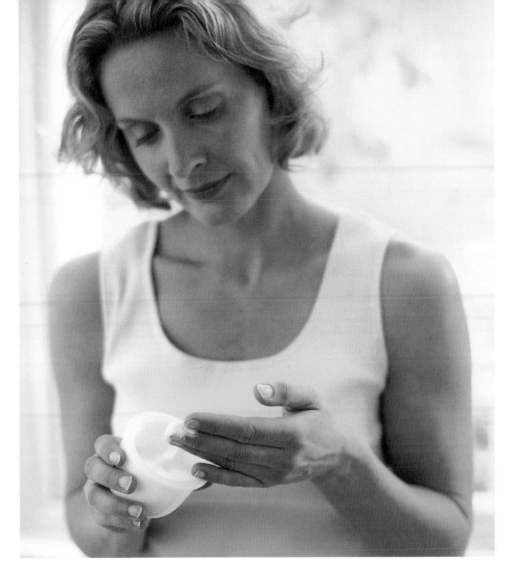

▷ **Roman chamomile is excellent for soothing dry, irritable and inflamed skin. Try adding a few drops to your moisturizer and apply daily.**

aromatherapy treatment

Aromatherapy can play an important part in the treatment of skin disorders. The oils are not only able to treat the physical symptoms but, through their aromas, can also affect the mental state of the sufferer. For example, many people suffering chronic, painful skin conditions, such as eczema and psoriasis, may have high stress levels because of the impact of the disease on their physical appearance.

Essential oils are able to break this cycle effectively, lightening the mind as well as tackling the physical symptoms. Where the skin is already being moisturized, whether on the face, hands and/or body, it is easy enough to combine appropriate essential oils with the existing treatment for a two-in-one effect. For example, arthritis oils added to a hand and body lotion base reduce pain and inflammation at the same time as making the skin less dry and scaly.

For severe eczema it is very beneficial to change your diet to one that is dairy-free, eliminating cow's milk and related products from what you eat. This is usually enough to cure the condition, although it can take a few months for the results to be evident. Meanwhile, correct use of the appropriate oils will bring relief from the symptoms.

Acne rosacea, a form of acne which usually attacks women over 30, has similar symptoms to *Acne vulgaris* (*see* The Teenage Years). It seems to affect women who like highly seasoned foods and drink large amounts of tea and coffee. Dietary changes will be highly beneficial in all cases, while the use of aromatherapy treatments will improve the condition of the skin.

Blending essential oils with a moisturizer

For customized skincare, select the appropriate essential oils and add them to a good quality, bland base cream. Add a little rose hip carrier oil if your skin is particularly dry.

ingredients
- 40 ml (8 tsp) unperfumed base cream
- rose hip oil (optional)
- blend of appropriate essential oils

equipment
- small jar
- swizzle stick or teaspoon
- spatula (optional)

tip

Always apply creams to the face with clean hands, and best of all using a spatula, to avoid transmitting germs from your fingernails to the cream, and possibly to your skin.

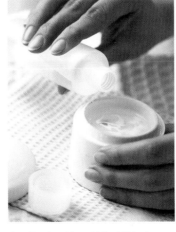

△ **1** For dry skin, add 5 ml (1 tsp) rose hip oil to a jar containing 40 ml (8 tsp) base moisturizing cream.

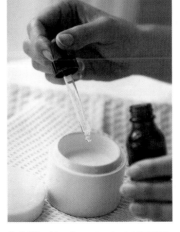

△ **2** After blending your own selection of appropriate essential oils, add 5 drops to the moisturizing cream.

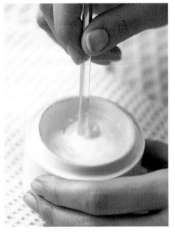

△ **3** Stir thoroughly with a swizzle stick or the handle of a clean teaspoon to blend the mixture.

Daily hand, foot and nail care

Our hands are exposed daily to the elements and to household detergents, and our feet carry us wherever we want to go. Both deserve as much attention as the face, and will benefit greatly from aromatherapy.

hand care

It is said that there are two ways to tell a woman's age: by her neck and by her hands. Our hands, like our necks and faces, are always exposed to the air and are always on visible display. However, it is easy to neglect them when leading a busy life.

treatment

Essential oils can be added to a base lotion and used after each time you wash your hands. Patchouli is one of the best oils for cracked, dry skin, and clary sage helps delay cellular aging. If your hands are neglected and in need of a boost, try giving them an exfoliating "mask" treatment before going to bed. After using an exfoliating face mask on your hands, apply your hand lotion. Cover your hands with cling film (plastic wrap) and pull on a pair of cotton gloves, or cotton socks, over the cling film. Keep the mask in place for an hour before rinsing off.

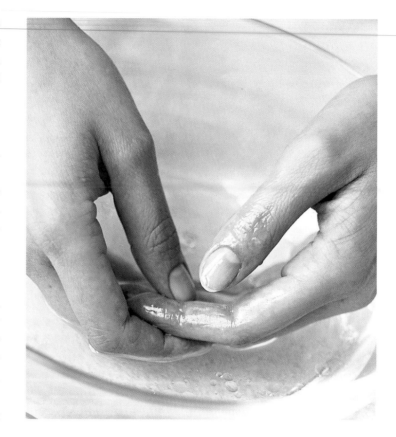

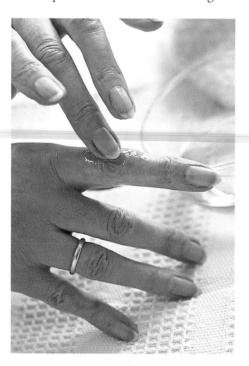

◁ For cracked knuckles, try patchouli oil mixed in a carrier cream or lotion base and applied to the affected area on clean, dry hands.

◁ **Having well-cared for hands is a beauty asset. To give your hands a treat, prepare a mix using oils of geranium and rose otto and work well into the skin.**

foot care

Think of the amount of work our feet have to do – we walk on them daily, often in inappropriate footwear, and yet we give them surprisingly little care and attention.

treatment

Spend some time each week giving your feet a treatment massage (*see* Swiss Reflex Therapy), which benefits your feet and the rest of your body at the same time. Keep them as scrupulously clean as your face, regularly removing dead skin at the heels and drying properly between the toes. Watch for any broken skin between the toes as this may be a sign of athlete's foot – a fungal condition which can be difficult to treat once it takes hold. Plastic shoes are a common cause of athlete's foot as they create moisture and cause the feet to sweat,

creating the ideal conditions for fungus to develop. Essential oils can be used to treat all fungus-type infections as well as viral ones, including warts and verrucas. You will also need to address the underlying causes. These may be related to stress and poor nutrition, and will be helped with relaxing essential oils.

nail care

Strong, well-manicured nails on the hands and feet play an important role in a woman's appearance. Brittle, damaged or weak nails can detract from this. Essential oils can be used to improve nail condition.

treatment

Essential oil of lavender is particularly good for strengthening nails. Each evening, put your finger on to the nozzle of a bottle of lavender oil, tip the bottle, and rub the oil into the cuticles. After two or three months you should see some improvement as the treated nail grows through.

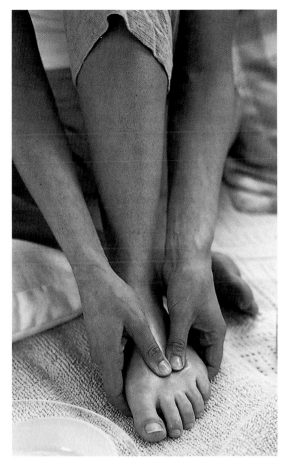

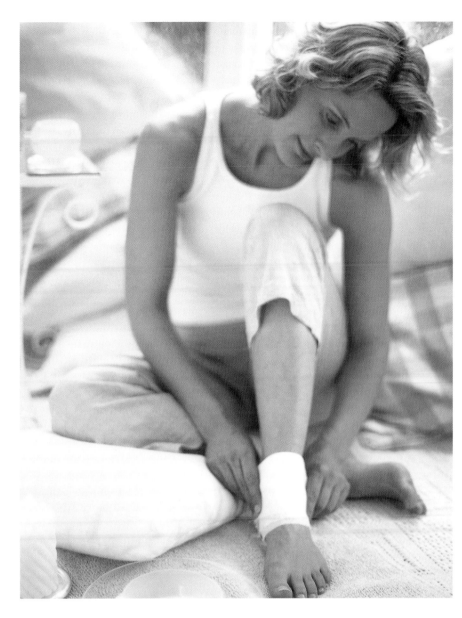

△ **Giving yourself a foot massage not only feels good but also energizes the many reflex points on your feet, which in turn correspond to different parts of the body.**

▷ **For tired or swollen ankles, a cool compress soaked in Roman chamomile and lavender oil is both soothing and refreshing and can also alleviate any inflammation.**

Nail treatment

Pampering your nails with this weekly treatment will keep them healthy and strong. If your nails are particularly weak and damaged, you may prefer to apply this quick treatment every evening. Because nail growth is a slow process, the results are not immediate – it will be a couple of months before you see any improvement, but it will be worth the wait.

ingredients
- warm water
- lavender essential oil

equipment
- bowl
- cuticle stick
- cotton bud (Q-tip)

tip

Sucking a jelly cube each day is said to stengthen the nails. If you often have white flecks across your nails, increasing the calcium in your diet could also help.

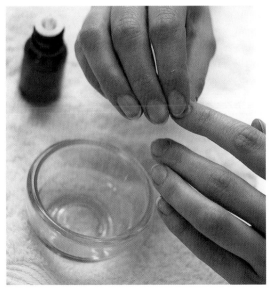

△ **1** Soak your fingertips in warm water before gently cleaning the surplus cuticle from the nails.

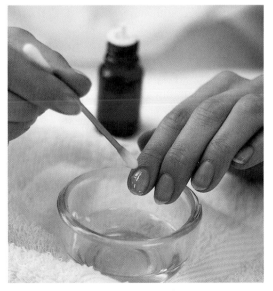

△ **2** Use a cotton bud (Q-tip) to apply neat lavender oil to each cuticle to strengthen them.

Daily bodycare

Our bodies are protected for much of the time with clothes, and because of this, the skin of our torso is usually in a better condition – softer and smoother – than that of our arms and legs, which are more frequently exposed to sunlight.

conditioning treatments

The arms and legs benefit hugely from the daily use of creams and lotions containing essential oils; improvements are particularly apparent when moisturizing bath or shower oils or gels have not been used as a matter of course. If your skin is dry or flaky, put your essential oils into a carrier oil to add a gleam to your skin. (*See* Preparing Oils for Application *to select the most beneficial oil for your skin type.*)

For a bath treatment for dry skin, grate 15 g (½ oz) unscented, non-alkaline soap into 120 ml (½ cup) boiling water, and stir to dissolve the soap. When cool, add 8 drops of your favourite essential oil or oil mix. Hold your mixture under the running tap to dissolve in the bathwater and make some bubbles. If you prefer lots of bubbles, add essential oils to a non-drying bubble bath.

If you have normal to oily skin, which is not known to be sensitive, give yourself a body rinse before leaving the bath or

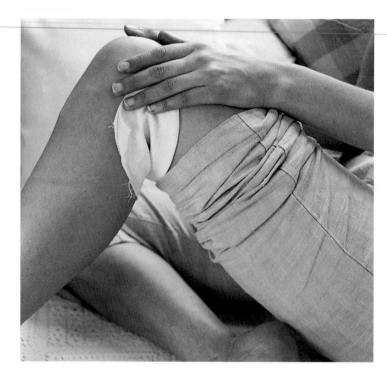

◁ Varicose veins can be painful and unsightly. A cool compress, made with cypress, clary sage or niaouli oil and applied to the affected area, can help.

shower. Dissolve your essential oil or oils into 15 ml (1 tbsp) vodka, and mix with 1 litre (1¾ pints) spring water. Add 120 ml (½ cup) white wine or cider vinegar to the spring water mixture for an extra zingy feel.

If you have a problem with body odour, use the vodka rinse above, but without the vinegar. Add 3 drops of nutmeg essential oil and 3 drops of cypress essential oil; both of these have deodorizing properties.

For hard, rough skin on elbows and heels, use a facial exfoliating mask, followed by a moisturizing body lotion or oil to which 2–3 drops of essential oil have been added.

Cellulite is caused by ineffective blood circulation, which leads to poor lymphatic drainage and fluid retention. Aromatherapy can help with a daily regime. Pummel the area vigorously before applying essential oils in a carrier lotion or oil.

Varicose vein treatment

Apply the essential oil blend or lotion mix to the whole leg before following the directions below. Upward strokes are important to help the blood move towards the heart. Use phlebotonic oils such as clary sage, cypress and niaouli.

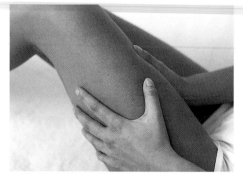

△ **1** Massage the upper half of the leg first with upward movements. This clears the valves to allow the blood to pass more easily from the lower leg.

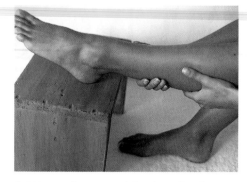

△ **2** Massage in an upward direction only, using the palms of both hands. Make long, firm strokes alternately with each hand up the calf muscle.

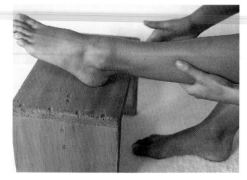

△ **3** Take the fingers of both hands alternately up the calf muscle. Complete the sequence by repeating step 2.

Anti-cellulite treatment

Cellulite is recognized by its resemblance to orange or grapefruit peel. A daily aromatherapy treatment, along with an improved diet and a thorough exercise plan, will boost the circulation and improve lymphatic drainage, helping to disperse the cellulite.

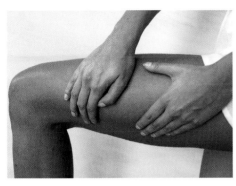

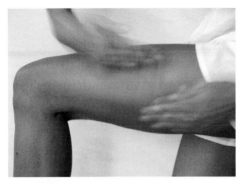

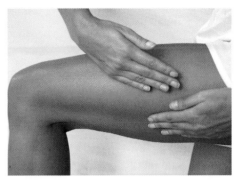

△ **1** After firmly rubbing in your prepared oil mix or lotion, take both hands alternately up the outside of the leg. Use a loofah or bristle brush if preferred.

△ **2** Use the heel of your hands to pummel the cellulite vigorously. This stimulates the circulation and allows quicker penetration of the essential oils.

△ **3** Continue to work over the cellulite area using the heels of both hands alternately. Maintaining the firmness of the strokes, repeat step 1.

Useful essential oils

essential oil	treatment
skin types	
DRY SKIN	
Chamomile (Roman) *Chamaemelum nobile*	anti-inflammatory (irritable skin)
Geranium *Pelargonium graveolens*	anti-infectious, cicatrizant
Lavender *Lavandula angustifolia*	antiseptic, anti-inflammatory, cicatrizant (healing)
Patchouli *Pogostemon patchouli*	anti-inflammatory, cicatrizant
Rose otto *Rosa damascena*	anti-inflammatory (blotchy skin), cicatrizant
OILY SKIN	
Cedarwood *Cedrus atlantica*	antiseptic, antibacterial, cicatrizant.
Lemon *Citrus limon*	astringent, antibacterial, anti-inflammatory
Ylang ylang *Cananga odorata*	tonic, balancing, calming, hypotensive
MATURE SKIN	
Clary sage *Salvia sclarea*	regenerative (cellular aging)
Frankincense *Boswellia carteri*	antioxidant (combats aging process), cicatrizant
anti-aging	
Clary sage *Salvia sclarea*	oestrogen-like, regenerative (counteracts cellular aging)
Frankincense *Boswellia carteri*	antioxidant (combats aging process)
Lemon *Citrus limon*	antisclerotic (combats aging process)

essential oil	treatment
skin conditions	
PSORIASIS (INCLUDING NAILS)	
Bergamot *Citrus bergamia*	cicatrizant
Lavender *Lavandula angustifolia*	cicatrizant
ECZEMA	
Bergamot *Citrus bergamia*	anti-infectious (weeping eczema), cicatrizant
Geranium *Pelargonium graveolens*	analgesic, anti-infectious, anti-inflammatory, cicatrizant
ACNE *ROSACEAE*	
Chamomile (German) *Matricaria recutica*	anti-inflammatory, cicatrizant
Chamomile (Roman) *Chamaemelum nobile*	anti-inflammatory, cicatrizant
Frankincense *Boswellia carteri*	analgesic, cicatrizant
ATHLETE'S FOOT AND NAIL FUNGI	
Clary sage *Salvia sclarea*	antifungal (skin conditions)
Geranium *Pelargonium graveolens*	antifungal, anti-infectious
Lavender *Lavandula angustifolia*	antifungal, antiseptic
CELLULITE	
Cypress *Cupressus sempervirens*	diuretic
Fennel *Foeniculum vulgare*	diuretic, circulatory stimulant
Juniper *Juniperus communis*	diuretic, lypolytic
VARICOSE VEINS	
See The Reproductive Years for relevant essential oils.	

Coping with stress

There is increasing evidence to suggest that stress features significantly in the lives of many women, whether they are single, married or co-habiting, and whether or not they have children. Many women are finding it increasingly difficult to manage work and home commitments, leisure time and relationships, and these stresses are often multiplied when a woman has children.

For many women, the workplace often provides the most anxiety because of the pressure to meet deadlines and performance targets and to succeed in today's economic jungle. For others, the home environment is full of tension and unresolved problems. Difficulties with a relationship, financial pressures, and/or troubles with children are problems which most women encounter at one point or another in their lives.

Perhaps stress can be defined as having too much to do, in too short a time, and without the necessary resources. When such a situation goes on and on over a period of time, it can have an adverse effect on health. When we are happy and contented, every cell in the body is influenced in a positive, life-affirming way, both emotionally and

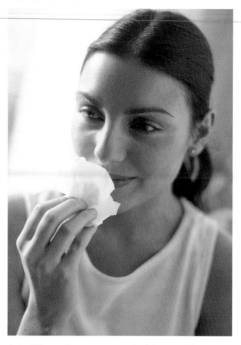

△ **Sniffing a tissue prepared with essential oils is a handy method for improving concentration.**

physically. However, when we are unhappy, or under too much pressure for an extended period of time, the cells generate a negative, health-reducing effect and stress-related conditions may begin to show: insomnia, tension headaches, chronic back problems,

digestive disorders, skin problems and other diseases in the body. Stress also affects our emotions, making us irritable and bad-tempered, and this intensifies problems in relationships with colleagues, friends and loved ones. It is a downward spiral that can eventually lead to clinical depression.

the use of aromatherapy

Essential oils have been proved to have an influence on the central nervous system, which varies depending on the essential oils selected. Good use of aromatherapy can improve general health and well-being, helping us to cope with the physical and emotional aspects of stress.

Stress can exacerbate PMS and other problems connected with menstruation. Conversely, difficult periods can increase stress levels. Essential oils can overcome these problems if they are used regularly.

Essential oils can work wonders to restore emotional health to a mind-body system that is out of balance. Used as part of a system of holistic care – so that the cause of the stress is dealt with – essential oils can offer much-needed relief. Often, this is all that is needed to break the negative cycle.

simple treatments

If you are finding it difficult to concentrate on your work, prepare a tissue with a blend of rosemary and peppermint essential oils, and sniff at intervals throughout the day. Both of these oils are decongestants and mental stimulants, and they should help to clear congested or conflicting thoughts and mixed emotions. Add lemon oil to the blend if you work on a computer. In one Japanese study, it was revealed that 54 per cent fewer typing errors were made by staff who had been exposed to a lemon aroma, compared to those who had not.

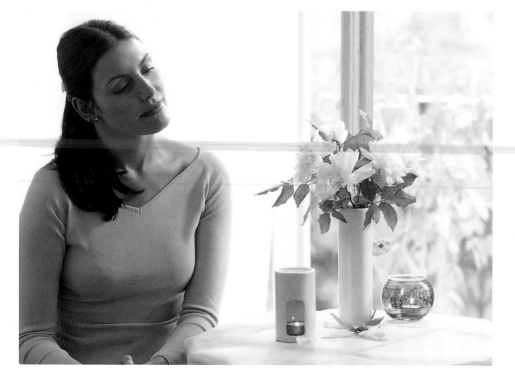

◁ **Inhalation is the fastest way for an essential oil to reach the brain. Vaporize ylang ylang for its balancing and calming properties.**

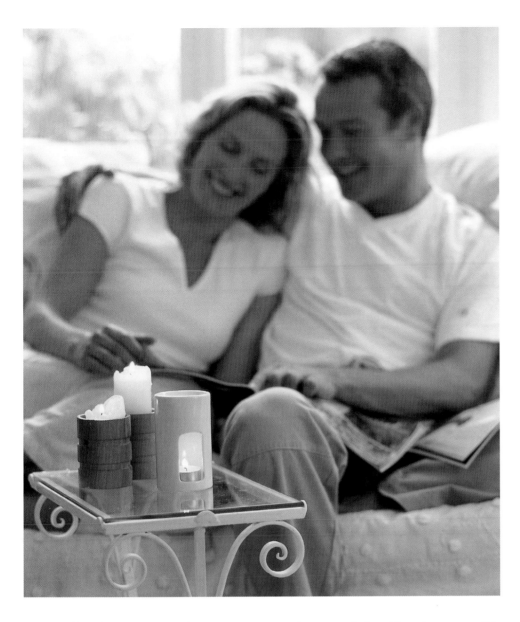

△ Juggling work and home commitments can place a strain on your relationship. Make sure you and your partner find enough time to relax together without being disturbed.

TIPS FOR COPING WITH STRESS

- Take regular exercise: join a gym, take up yoga, or go for long walks.
- Put aside some quiet time each day for yourself, for reading, reflection, meditation, visiting friends, or simply doing nothing at all.
- Eat a healthy diet, avoiding the temptation to snack on processed foods, even when you think you don't have time for meals.
- Devise a schedule at home which means that everyone takes part in running the household.
- If you have a partner, make sure you spend at least one evening a week on your own together.
- Unwind in an aromatherapy bath with a favourite essential oil every evening: this promotes a refreshing sleep, which will help to prepare you for the next day.

The effect that an aroma can have on our emotions depends to an extent on whether or not we like the smell, and whether it holds any positive or negative associations for us. The interpretation of an aroma is a very individual matter and it is difficult to forecast the effect it will have on any one person. The limbic system, where aromas are interpreted, is said to be responsible for our sexuality, our impulses of attraction and aversion, our motivation, moods, and memory, and also our creativity. It is the combination of all of these things that makes us unique as individuals. Finding the aromas that really work for you is often a matter of trial and error.

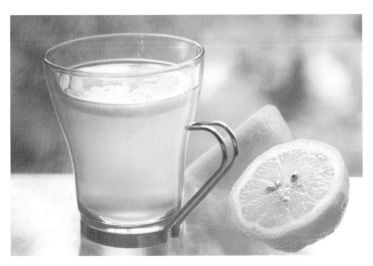

△ Lemon rind (zest) contains the essential oil of lemon. Put a slice into water for an uplifting drink.

▷ Lank, lifeless hair may be an early sign of stress. Roman chamomile added to your hair conditioner can restore shine and also calm your nerves.

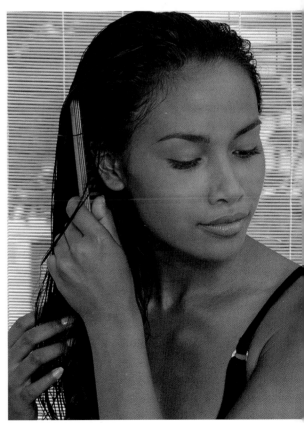

Emotional insecurity

The emotions we express or feel can be separated into two groups: primary and secondary. Some primary emotions are positive, such as feelings of love, tolerance, and happiness, and these are not a problem. Difficulties arise with the negative primary emotions, such as fear, anger, guilt and jealousy. Secondary emotions are usually concerned with our personality. These may be shown as moodiness, confusion, timidity and inferiority, for example.

Essential oils are very useful for treating emotional problems. The oils are selected on the basis of their properties which relate to the emotion being expressed. For example, essential oils which have relaxing and anti-inflammatory properties are known to be soothing for anger, while oils with stimulating and digestive properties are better able to overcome fear.

anger

The state of anger can range from mild irritability and impatience at one end of the scale to explosive outbursts and fury at the other. The ability to cope with anger varies from person to person, depending on the personality. When under stress, anger is more easily aroused and our ability to deal with our own feelings may be severely tested. It is important to have the ability to come to terms with our own anger and to handle it in a positive, constructive way. Otherwise, we may jeopardize both professional and personal relationships. The oils which help are, principally, calming, anti-spasmodic, anti-inflammatory and healing.

fear

Stress and fear are sometimes related, and can be acute or chronic. If you oversleep and are running late for an important meeting, for example, your body goes into a temporary state of fear and your adrenal glands produce extra adrenalin to help you deal with the situation. However, if the state of fear is long-lasting, it can become a chronic condition that can lead to illness. As an example, some people worry about money, not necessarily because they don't have enough, but because they fear that bad times lie ahead, so they save compulsively and are afraid to enjoy the money they have. Living in a state of fear creates tension and anxiety which have a detrimental effect on our outlook and upon our bodies. The helpful essential oils are those which are analgesic, calming and soothing, and those which are stimulating to the mind, as well as to the respiratory and digestive systems.

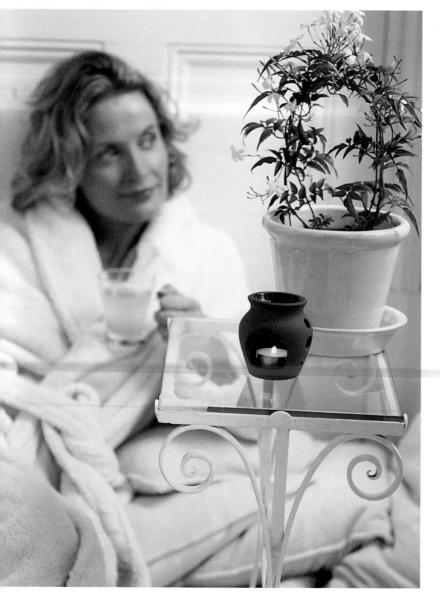

◁ **After a difficult day or an emotional upset, give yourself time to sit quietly and recover. Geranium, lavender and lemon are helpful for angry or jealous outbursts. Try a few drops in a vaporizer an hour before bedtime.**

▷ **Our sleep pattern can be disturbed by a negative emotional state. Sprinkle a few drops of undiluted lavender oil on to a tissue and place this inside your pillowslip for a peaceful night's sleep.**

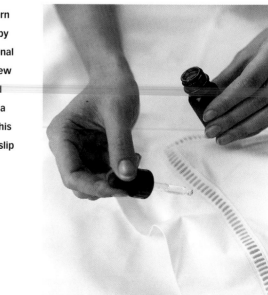

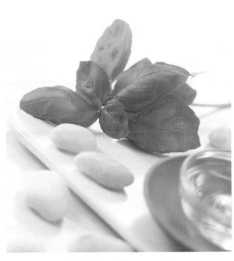

△ **Basil is useful for its effects on the nervous system. It can help to dispel fear and jealousy.**

jealousy

Most jealous feelings are negative. Jealousy is often linked with anger and/or resentment, and may arise out of an inability to share our friends, family and possessions, or else out of a craving for things that we do not have, which other people (particularly those around us) seem to have. A woman may covet her friend's physical attributes, her successful career, or her conflict-free partnership. Although jealousy is often the most difficult emotion to admit to, it is one of the most deadly, where we stand to hurt not only others but also ourselves. Positive thinking and the use of essential oils which will detoxify or destroy fungi and kill viruses can help to overcome this self-destructive emotion.

Secondary emotions can also be helped by essential oils and are sometimes linked with a primary emotion like fear. Lack of

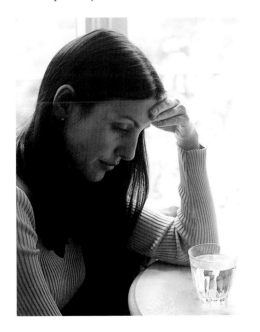

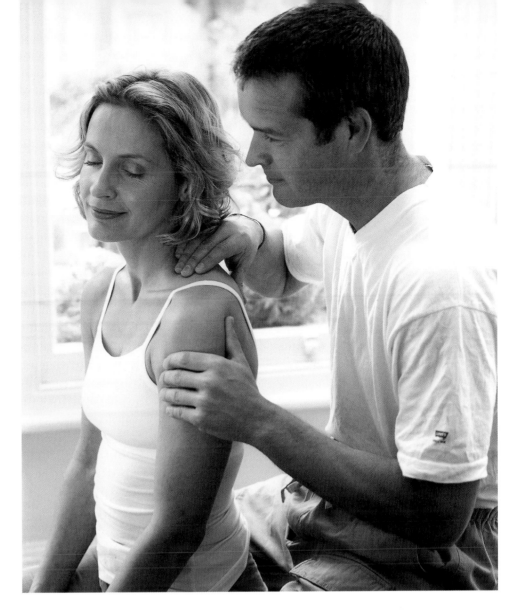

△ **A shoulder massage using juniper oil can help when you are feeling emotionally drained.**

confidence or a sense of under-achievement may involve fear, and mood swings may involve anger and/or irritability.

lack of confidence

Many women suffer from a lack of self-confidence. It can be difficult for women who return to work after being at home bringing up children, or for a woman who is working with people to whom she feels (or is made to feel) inferior. Positive thinking is necessary here, along with neurotonic essential oils which will boost your morale by strengthening the nervous system. These stimulate the mind and will help you to achieve things you never thought were possible. Sweet thyme may help to promote bravery and instil drive and assertiveness due to its many tonic properties. The most effective methods of use are by tissue or vaporizer inhalation, and in the bath.

◁ **Water with lemon and peppermint can help to dispel apathy and lift feelings of depression.**

moodiness

As well as being able to relax or stimulate the nervous system, essential oils can also induce slight mood changes. This makes the use of essential oils suitable for women who are inclined to be temperamental, and for the unpredictable mood swings and irritability suffered during PMS.

loss of sensual awareness

Feelings of indifference, apathy and general loss of libido can be directly related to stress and/or overwork. Taking an essential oil bath or vaporizing some oils an hour before bedtime will help you to unwind, physically and emotionally. You and your partner may like to give each other aromatherapy back or shoulder massages to help each other relax and to prepare for love-making. Use essential oils which are renowned for their aphrodisiac and uplifting effects.

Common health problems

beauty and well-being

There are several relatively common health problems which can occur at any age and with varying degrees of severity. Stress generally makes all these conditions worse.

irritable bowel syndrome (IBS)

This disorder of the lower bowel usually occurs between 20-40 years of age. The usual symptoms are colicky pains, diarrhoea and/or constipation, and distension of the abdomen, giving rise to noisy rumblings and wind. Emotional factors can play an important part in this disorder, and those who are anxious and over-conscientious are the most likely sufferers. Symptoms can be worse just before a period, especially if PMS is present.

It is useful to experiment with diet. Exclude cow's milk and its products and monitor the result. Foods which contain wheat can also cause problems, as can the caffeine in tea and coffee. Try essential oils which balance the digestive system, used in a variety of ways: by ingestion (*see* Aromatherapy Techniques), by application of oils in a carrier base, rubbed on to the abdomen twice daily in a clockwise direction, and by compresses placed over the abdomen.

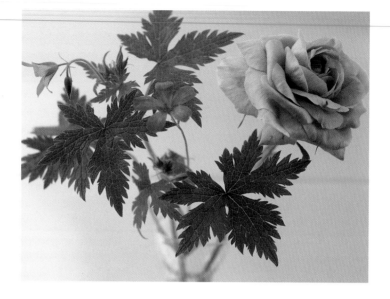

◁ **The heady yet gentle aroma of rose is a favourite with almost every woman. Rose helps to lift the spirits and promote feelings of well-being.**

cystitis

This is a common problem that can occur after sex and during pregnancy. Cystitis is an infection and inflammation of the bladder and urethra. It is characterized by a frequent, painful urge to go to the toilet. Treatment is with antibacterial and antiseptic essential oils which have an affinity to the kidneys. Cystitis has been treated successfully using a tea with the relevant essential oils added (*see* Aromatherapy Techniques) and by application of the same oils in a carrier base to the abdomen and lower back.

sinusitis

Inflammation of the sinus area around the nose and/or eyes can occur at any time in life after puberty and is often difficult to cure, even with an operation. It causes chronic congestion, catarrh and sometimes headaches. Fortunately, sinusitis can be helped easily and successfully by adding the appropriate essential oils to your regular moisturizer. Allergic reactions or colds can exacerbate the condition, in which case neat essential oils should be inhaled on a tissue or used in the bath. Pressing on the sinus-pressure points on the feet (*see* Swiss Reflex Therapy) every night while symptoms persist is also helpful.

vaginitis

Inflammation of the vagina, with accompanying irritation, can be caused by leaving a tampon in too long or through use of the contraceptive pill. The most frequent cause is when a yeast-like substance, called *Candida albicans*, a normal inhabitant of the mouth and bowel (and, in women, of the vagina) becomes infected. When symptoms first appear, immediate treatment with essential oils will help. Provided a tampon was not the cause of the inflammation in the first place, try a tampon with 2 drops of tea tree oil inserted into the vagina and left in

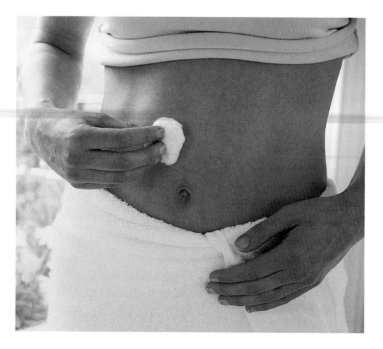

▷ **An application of fennel, peppermint and/or rosemary can be helpful with IBS. Use in a carrier oil or compress applied to the abdomen area.**

overnight. Alternatively, taking regular sitz-baths for ten minutes at a time, using a synergistic mix of appropriate essential oils, can also help.

thrush

Infected *Candida albicans* can show as white ulcerous spots inside the mouth (thrush), which can be dealt with using a mouthwash including anti-infectious essential oils. The vagina can also be affected with thrush, giving rise to itching and discomfort. Thrush usually affects women with a low immune system, where it can be due to stress, the overuse of antibiotics or diabetes. Additional symptoms which can present themselves at this time include cystitis, depression and headaches.

With thrush it is helpful if the intake of sugar and refined carbohydrates in the diet is reduced immediately. If the condition worsens, an effective form of aromatherapy treatment involves eating live yogurt containing suitable essential oils: 20 drops of oil to 100 ml (6-7 tbsp) of yogurt and, if possible, inserting some of this mixture into the vagina with a tampon applicator.

endometriosis

This condition is when tissue similar to that of the lining of the uterus is found else-where – mostly in the ovaries. The tissue swells and bleeds, causing severe pain before a period and excessive blood loss during it. Conventional treatment may recommend removal of the ovaries (and therefore the

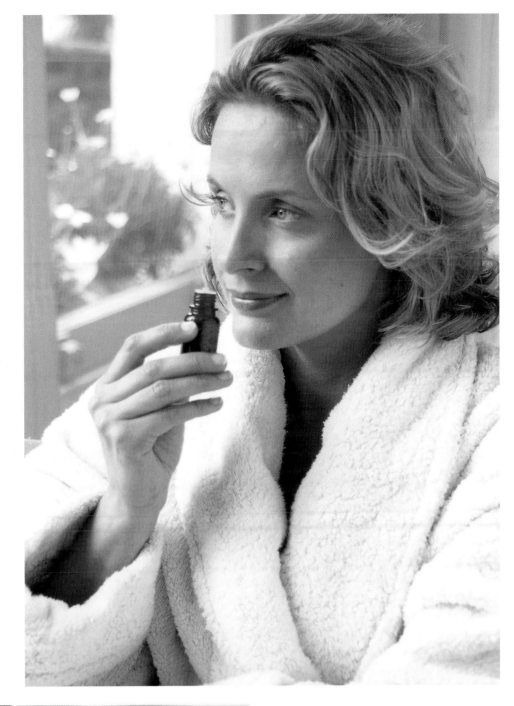

△ **Peppermint is useful for relieving nasal congestion and treating general sinus problems**.

hormone production) so that the uterus is no longer stimulated to produce the extra tissue. The contraceptive pill is often prescribed but this is not always successful.

Some women prefer to avoid surgery if possible, in which case it is worth trying hormone-like and decongestant essential oils first, as they have been known to help. If surgery is inevitable, then oestrogen-like essential oils will help the body to readjust itself to the loss of the ovaries.

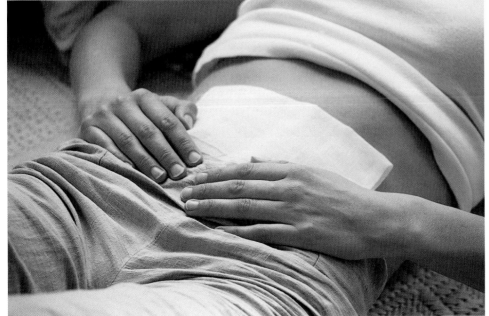

◁ **A compress of clary sage and cypress can be used for problems associated with the ovaries**.

Useful essential oils

essential oil	treatment
stress	
Chamomile (Roman) *Chamaemelum nobile*	calming
Lemon *Citrus limon*	calming, hypotensive
Melissa *Melissa officinalis*	calming, sedative
Ylang ylang *Cananga odorata*	balancing, calming, hypotensive
depression	
Basil *Ocimum basilicum* var. *album*	neurotonic
Frankincense *Boswellia carteri*	energizing, immunostimulant
Juniper *Juniperus communis*	neurotonic
Neroli *Citrus aurantium* var. *amara*	tranquilizing (nervous depression, fatigue)
Niaouli *Melaleuca viridiflora*	tonic
Peppermint *Mentha* x *piperita*	neurotonic
Pine *Pinus sylvestris*	neurotonic
Rosemary *Rosmarinus officinalis*	neurotonic, sexual tonic
stress with depression	
Bergamot *Citrus bergamia*	balancing, calming, sedative, tonic to central nervous system
Clary sage *Salvia sclarea*	balancing, relaxing, neurotonic
Cypress *Cupressus sempervirens*	balancing, calming, neurotonic
Geranium *Pelargonium graveolens*	balancing, relaxing, stimulant (nervous fatigue)
Lavender *Lavandula angustifolia*	balancing, calming, sedative, tonic
Marjoram *Origanum majorana*	balancing, calming, neurotonic
Rose otto *Rosa damascena*	balancing, relaxing, neurotonic, sexual tonic
poor concentration	
Basil *Ocimum basilicum* var. *album*	neurotonic
Bergamot *Citrus bergamia*	balancing, tonic
Thyme (sweet) *Thymus vulgaris*	cardiotonic, neurotonic, immunostimulant
irritable bowel syndrome	
Fennel *Foeniculum vulgare*	analgesic, antispasmodic, digestive (constipation, diarrhoea, flatulence)
Peppermint *Mentha* x *piperita*	analgesic, anti-inflammatory, digestive (diarrhoea, flatulence)
Rosemary *Rosmarinus officinalis*	analgesic, antispasmodic, digestive (constipation, flatulence)

essential oil	treatment
thrush (*Candida albicans*) and vaginitis	
Lavender *Lavandula angustifolia*	analgesic, antifungal, anti-inflammatory
Pine *Pinus sylvestris*	analgesic, antifungal, anti-infectious, anti-inflammatory, neurotonic
Tea tree *Melaleuca alternifolia*	analgesic, antifungal, anti-infectious, anti-inflammatory, immunostimulant, neurotonic
Thyme (sweet) *Thymus vulgaris*	antifungal, anti-infectious, anti-inflammatory, immunostimulant, neurotonic
cystitis	
Eucalyptus *Eucalyptus smithii*	anti-infectious, antiseptic
Juniper *Juniperus communis*	anti-inflammatory, antiseptic
Lavender *Lavandula angustifolia*	anti-inflammatory, antiseptic
Thyme (sweet) *Thymus vulgaris*	anti-infectious, anti-inflammatory, antiseptic
sinusitis	
Eucalyptus *Eucalyptus smithii*	anti-inflammatory, antiseptic
Lavender *Lavandula angustifolia*	anti-inflammatory, anti-infectious, antiseptic
Peppermint *Mentha* x *piperita*	anti-inflammatory, anti-infectious
endometriosis	
Clary sage *Salvia sclarea*	decongestant, oestrogen-like, phlebotonic
Cypress *Cupressus sempervirens*	astringent, hormone-like (ovary problems), phlebotonic
Geranium *Pelargonium graveolens*	analgesic, astringent, cicatrizant, decongestant, phlebotonic, styptic
Rose otto *Rosa damascena*	astringent, cicatrizant, neurotonic, styptic

Sweet scents are the swift vehicles

of still sweeter thoughts.

Walter Savage Landor, 1775–1864.

essential oil	treatment

anger, fear and jealousy

The following essential oils given can benefit all of these emotions. The properties required for each condition are listed first, the oils which follow show the properties each possesses relevant to that particular emotion.

ANGER

Look for oils which are	analgesic, anticatarrhal, anti-inflammatory, antispasmodic, calming, carminative (relieving flatulence), cicatrizant, sedative
Basil *Ocimum basilicum* var. *album*	analgesic, anti-inflammatory, carminative, calming to the nervous system
Bergamot *Citrus bergamia*	antispasmodic, calming, cicatrizant
Geranium *Pelargonium graveolens*	analgesic, anti-inflammatory, antispasmodic, cicatrizant, relaxant
Juniper *Juniperus communis*	analgesic, anticatarrhal, anti-inflammatory
Lavender *Lavandula angustifolia*	analgesic, anti-inflammatory, antispasmodic, calming and sedative, cicatrizant
Lemon *Citrus limon*	anti-inflammatory, antispasmodic, calming, carminative

FEAR

Look for oils which are	antispasmodic, cardiotonic, calming and soothing, digestive, hypotensive, mental stimulant, nausea relief, nerve tonic, respiratory tonic, sedative
Basil *Ocimum basilicum* var. *album*	antispasmodic, cardiotonic, neurotonic
Bergamot *Citrus bergamia*	antispasmodic (indigestion), calming, sedative (agitation), nerve tonic
Geranium *Pelargonium graveolens*	antispasmodic, relaxant
Juniper *Juniperus communis*	digestive tonic, nerve tonic
Lavender *Lavandula angustifolia*	antispasmodic, calming, cardiotonic, hypotensive, sedative
Lemon *Citrus limon*	antispasmodic (diarrhoea normalizing), calming, hypotensive, nausea relief

The flowers anew, returning seasons bring

But beauty faded has no second spring.

From The First Pastoral, Ambrose Philips, 1675–1749.

essential oil	treatment

JEALOUSY

Look for oils which are	antibacterial, antifungal, antiviral, cicatrizant, detoxifying, litholytic
Basil *Ocimum basilicum* var. *album*	antibacterial, antiviral, decongestant (uterine)
Bergamot *Citrus bergamia*	antibacterial, antiviral, cicatrizant
Geranium *Pelargonium graveolens*	antibacterial, antifungal, cicatrizant, decongestant (lymph)
Juniper *Juniperus communis*	detoxifying, litholytic
Lavender *Lavandula angustifolia*	antibacterial, antifungal, cicatrizant
Lemon *Citrus limon*	antibacterial, antifungal, antiviral, litholytic

irritability

Chamomile (Roman) *Chamaemelum nobile*	calming
Cypress *Cupressus sempervirens*	calming
Rose otto *Rosa damascena*	calming

lack of confidence

Basil *Ocimum basilicum* var. *album*	neurotonic
Bergamot *Citrus bergamia*	balancing, tonic to central nervous system
Lavender *Lavandula angustifolia*	balancing, tonic
Marjoram *Origanum majorana*	balancing, neurotonic
Rosemary *Rosmarinus officinalis*	neurotonic
Thyme (sweet) *Thymus vulgaris*	cardiotonic, neurotonic, immunostimulant

Sensual awareness

Ylang ylang *Cananga odorata*	reproductive stimulant (frigidity, impotence)
Rose otto *Rosa damascena*	sexual tonic (frigidity, sexual debility)

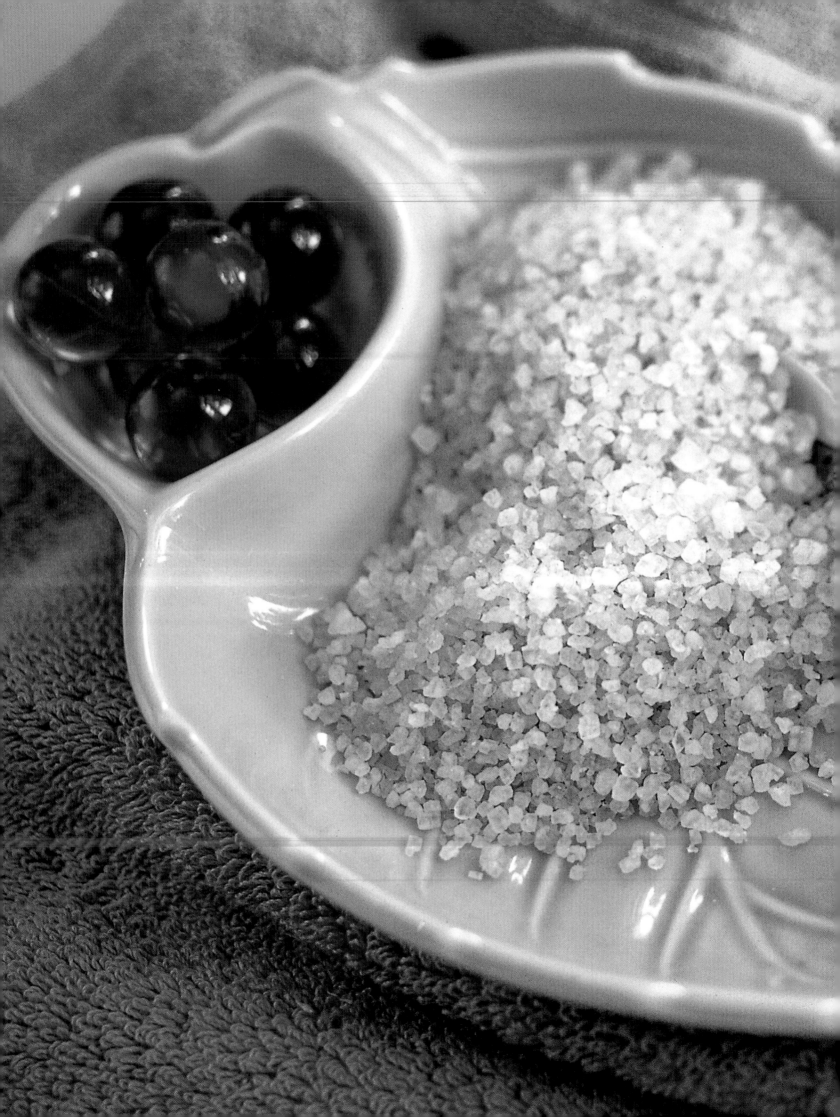

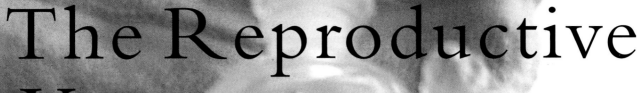

The Reproductive Years

For you created me in my mother's womb.
I praise you because I am fearfully and
wonderfully made.

From Psalm 139:13, The Holy Bible.

Coping with menstruation

When a girl reaches puberty, her previously dormant ovaries begin to release eggs for potential fertilization in the uterus. The ovaries take it in turns, approximately once a month, to release one, or sometimes two, eggs. The length of this cycle varies between individuals, from three to five weeks on average. The menstrual cycle is controlled by several hormones released by the endocrine system: these include oestrogen and progesterone, the latter being responsible for the thickening of the uterus lining, ready to welcome and feed a fertilized egg. At the same time, the breasts begin to swell a little, as they prepare to produce milk-forming tissue, and congestion occurs, particularly in the area between the nipples and the armpits.

If the egg is not fertilized within a few days, it dies and, together with the lining of the uterus, is rejected by the uterus two weeks after its arrival. The result is a flow of blood lasting, on average, between three and five days. Once finished, it can take up to three weeks before the next egg is released, depending on the individual.

This hormonal activity can cause period pain (dysmenorrhoea), irregularity, a heavy blood flow (menorrhagia), hardly

▷ **For some women, their periods are marked by a dull backache. Sweet marjoram, rosemary and pine can be applied on a warm compress to the painful area.**

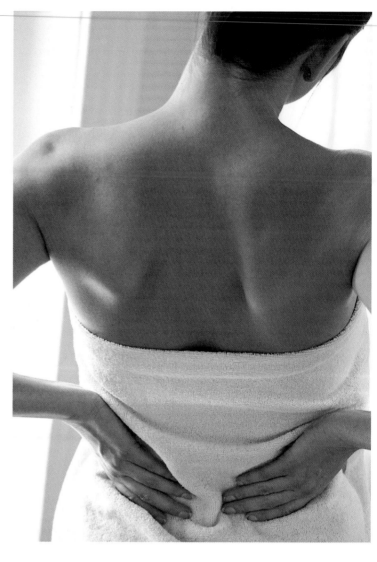

△ **Peppermint is useful for treating nausea and headaches. It can be taken internally in water.**

any flow (oligomenorrhoea) or perhaps no flow at all (amenorrhoea). Other symptoms may appear, and can vary from water retention, constipation, backache, tiredness, nausea, headaches and migraine, to tender breasts and premenstrual syndrome (PMS). This emotional complication of PMS can adversely affect the rest of the family as well as the sufferer. PMS should not be confused with period pains or any of the other symptoms experienced during menstruation, as the moment blood flow begins, PMS symptoms disappear.

painful periods

These are caused by congestion of blood in the uterus. Symptoms can range from a slight discomfort to a heavy, dragging pain in the abdomen. For some women, period pains may also affect the lower back.

treatment

Apply analgesic and decongestant essential oils in a vegetable oil or lotion carrier-base, in a clockwise direction, over the entire abdomen, daily at bedtime, eight to ten days before your period is due. When you have pain or tender breasts it is beneficial to apply a warm compress, using the same essential oils as above (*see* Aromatherapy Techniques). Exercise can be helpful as it stimulates the blood circulation and relieves congestion. After childbirth, period pains usually diminish or disappear.

irregular, infrequent or lack of periods

This can be very frustrating from the point of view of planning your life, especially if you are trying to conceive a child. The problem is due to hormonal imbalance. Worry can make things worse, so stress-relieving essential oils, when used regularly, can be beneficial.

treatment

Roman chamomile, melissa and rose otto essential oils can be blended together in a carrier-base oil or lotion and rubbed into the abdomen, in a clockwise direction. The appropriate, hormone-like, essential oils should also be used.

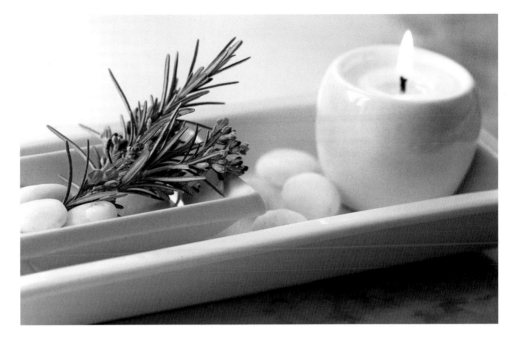

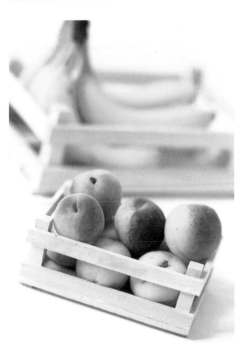

scanty and heavy periods

These may be due to an imbalance of prostaglandin in the body, a hormone which affects the uterus. With heavy periods, the lining of the uterus is over-thick.

treatment

Use hormone-like essential oils.

other symptoms

Constipation, tiredness and backache can all arise as a result of period problems. Other

△ **Rosemary is a good choice to help with period problems, relieving constipation and fatigue.**

symptoms which can arise around the time of menstruation are associated with PMS.

treatment

Many oils are effective against backache, and it is probably best to experiment until you find the ones you like best. Rosemary and mandarin, used together, are known to be effective for constipation.

◁ **Include plenty of fresh fruit in your daily diet. Healthy eating can alleviate period problems.**

LIFESTYLE TIPS FOR MENSTRUAL PROBLEMS

- Foods to avoid: excess sugar, salt, chocolate
- Foods to eat: liver, fish, fresh fruit (especially bananas), nuts, pulses, raw or cooked fresh vegetables (especially greens), salads (with evening primrose oil), diuretic vegetables, such as fennel, cucumber and cabbage (try cooking cabbage in a minimum amount of water and drink the water that is left after cooking).
- Drinks to avoid: excess caffeine found in tea, coffee and cola.

▷ **Experiment with making your own lotions. Choose the oils most suited to your symptoms and have a bottle made up and ready to use.**

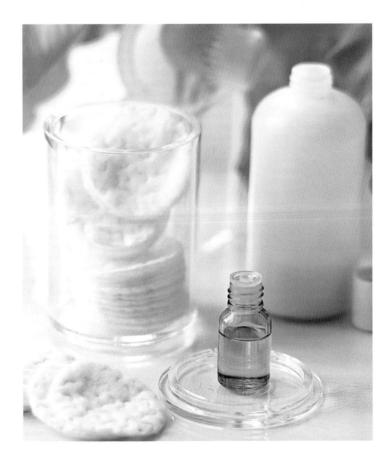

Pre-menstrual syndrome (PMS)

Some researchers estimate that PMS affects up to half of adult women living in modern society. No one knows exactly the cause of PMS, but it is believed that the lowered hormone level in the body after the egg has been released is mainly responsible for the collection of mental and physical symptoms which can become apparent eight to ten days before menstruation. Contributory factors include poor nutrition and stress: women often juggle many responsibilities at the same time, with insufficient time to eat properly and relax.

excessive water retention

Fluid retention is thought to be a crucial factor in PMS, as it affects all the cells in the body. PMS may be accompanied by weight gain and shows itself in the swelling of the abdomen, ankles and breasts, which can become very tender and swollen.

treatment

Diuretic and decongestant essential oils can be used to help reduce swelling.

persistent headaches and sleep disturbances

Both a lack of sleep and regular headaches are draining on the body, and will increase stress levels and the inability to cope.

treatment

Calming, neurotonic and decongestant essential oils can be used to relieve the headaches and/or insomnia by balancing the whole body.

emotional instability

Many women suffer from depression and irritability every month. In some cases, this can be severe and can lead to arguments and difficulties at home and at work.

treatment

Antidepressive and calming essential oils, taken as inhalations and baths, can help.

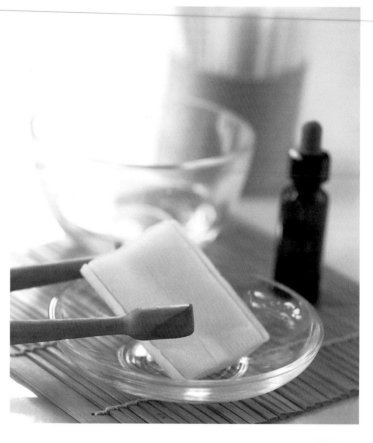

◁ **To make a compress, add a few drops of your chosen oil blend to a bowl of water and mix well. Place a piece of cloth on the water's surface and let the oil soak into it. Use as needed.**

▽ **For sleepless nights, headaches, and irritability prepare a mix of Roman chamomile, melissa and lavender. It may be handy to keep some by your bedside.**

LIFESTYLE TIPS FOR PMS

For the most effective results, a holistic approach to PMS is essential.

- Amend your diet to boost your general health and vitality
- Exercise to stimulate your blood circulation and to relieve congestion: try walking, cycling and swimming.
- Avoid stressful situations wherever possible, and ask for help if home or work responsibilities become too much
- Take your favourite relevant essential oils to work for instant therapy

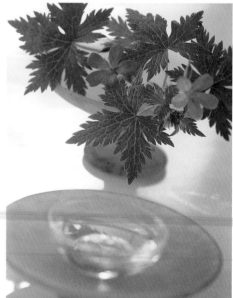

hormonal treatment

Some essential oils have a tendency to normalize hormonal secretions, including those involved in the reproductive system. Cypress is helpful for all ovarian problems. Clary sage and niaouli are oestrogen-like, which makes them useful for the stages in a woman's life when oestrogen production is unstable. To balance your hormones, these oils should be used in applications, baths and inhalations ten to 12 days before the expected start of a period.

Useful essential oils

essential oil	treatment

hormone-like essential oils

essential oil	treatment
Chamomile (German) *Matricaria recutica*	decongestant, hormone-like
Clary sage *Salvia sclarea*	decongestant, oestrogen-like
Cypress *Cupressus sempervirens*	hormone-like (ovarian)
Niaouli *Melaleuca viridiflora*	oestrogen-like (regularizes menses)
Peppermint *Mentha* x *piperita*	hormone-like (ovarian stimulant), neurotonic

painful periods and backache

essential oil	treatment
Basil *Ocimum basilicum* var. *album*	analgesic, antispasmodic, decongestant
Eucalyptus *Eucalyptus smithii* (not *Eucalyptus globulus*)	analgesic, decongestant
Geranium *Pelargonium graveolens*	analgesic, antispasmodic, decongestant
Lavender *Lavandula angustifolia*	analgesic, antispasmodic, calming, sedative, tonic
Marjoram (sweet) *Origanum majorana*	analgesic, antispasmodic, calming, neurotonic
Peppermint *Mentha* x *piperita*	analgesic, decongestant, hormone-like (ovarian stimulant)
Pine *Pinus sylvestris*	analgesic, decongestant
Rosemary *Rosmarinus officinalis*	analgesic, antispasmodic, decongestant

irregular, scanty and/or lack of periods

Mix a blend using the hormone-like essential oils (above). Other possibilities include:

essential oil	treatment
Chamomile (Roman) *Chamaemelum nobile*	calming, menstrual regulator, nervous menstrual problems
Melissa *Melissa officinalis*	calming, sedative, regularizes secretions
Rose otto *Rosa damascena*	general reproductive system regulator

heavy periods

essential oil	treatment
Cypress *Cupressus sempervirens*	astringent, phlebotonic, hormone-like (ovary problems)
Melissa *Melissa officinalis*	calming, sedative, regularizes secretions

fluid retention

essential oil	treatment
Cypress *Cupressus sempervirens*	diuretic (oedema, rheumatic swelling)
Fennel *Foeniculum vulgare*	diuretic (cellulite, oedema)
Juniper *Juniperus communis*	diuretic (cellulite, oedema)
Sage *Salvia officinalis*	decongestant, lypolytic (cellulite)

low spirits (depression) and fatigue

essential oil	treatment
Basil *Ocimum basilicum* var. *album*	nervous system regulator (anxiety), neurotonic (convalescence, depression)
Chamomile (Roman) *Chamaemelum nobile*	calming (nervous depression, nervous shock)
Clary sage *Salvia sclarea*	neurotonic (nervous fatigue)
Geranium *Pelargonium graveolens*	relaxant (anxiety, debility, nervous fatigue)
Juniper *Juniperus communis*	neurotonic (debility, fatigue)
Marjoram (sweet) *Origanum majorana*	neurotonic (debility, mental instability, anguish, nervous depression)
Pine *Pinus sylvestris*	neurotonic (debility, fatigue)
Rosemary *Rosmarinus officinalis*	neurotonic (general debility and fatigue)

tender, congested breasts

essential oil	treatment
Eucalyptus *Eucalyptus smithii* (not *Eucalyptus globulus*)	analgesic, decongestant
Geranium *Pelargonium graveolens*	analgesic, decongestant

headaches

essential oil	treatment
Chamomile (Roman) *Chamaemelum nobile*	antispasmodic, calming, sedative
Lavender *Lavandula angustifolia*	analgesic, calming, sedative
Marjoram (sweet) *Origanum majorana*	analgesic, antispasmodic, calming
Melissa *Melissa officinalis*	calming, sedative
Peppermint *Mentha* x *piperita*	analgesic, antispasmodic
Rosemary *Rosmarinus officinalis*	analgesic, antispasmodic, decongestant

insomnia

essential oil	treatment
Basil *Ocimum basilicum* var. *album*	nervous system regulator (nervous insomnia)
Chamomile (Roman) *Chamaemelum nobile*	calming, sedative
Lavender *Lavandula angustifolia*	calming, sedative
Lemon *Citrus limon*	calming
Melissa *Melissa officinalis*	calming, sedative

irritability

essential oil	treatment
Chamomile (Roman) *Chamaemelum nobile*	calming, sedative

Preparing for pregnancy

Once the menstrual cycle begins, becoming pregnant is a possibility until periods end at the menopause. Once an egg is fertilized, the body's hormones begin to change and can give rise to many symptoms, some of which can be helped with essential oils.

after conception

A normal pregnancy lasts approximately nine months. It is divided into three periods of approximately three months, known as trimesters. Once you realize that you are pregnant, you may experience a variety of emotions, ranging from joy and delight to fear and apprehension. Towards the end of the first trimester your breasts may feel tender and your appetite may increase. At this stage you may develop a heightened sense of smell, and this may start to affect your food preferences.

The second trimester is probably the most enjoyable, as you gradually become accustomed to the physical and emotional aspects of having a baby. During this time, you can benefit from using essential oils to help with some of the stresses and strains you may be experiencing as you adjust to the changes that are taking place in your body. Remember that any essential oils you use for yourself will also reach your baby, and they should be used with care and common sense if you are both to reap the benefits.

By the third trimester you will look well and truly pregnant and your body will start to feel heavy and cumbersome. During this time you need more rest, preferably with your feet up, and you will be starting to make preparations for labour.

Throughout the pregnancy be sure to eat well. You also need to look after your teeth: your baby will take from you whatever nutrition he or she needs and it is you who will be deprived of essential nutrients such as calcium and iron. Listen to your body: a food craving can often indicate your baby's and your own body's needs. For example, a craving for cheese could mean your body needs more calcium and protein.

cautions during pregnancy

You may not know you are pregnant until two months have already passed. If you are trying to conceive, you should use only the

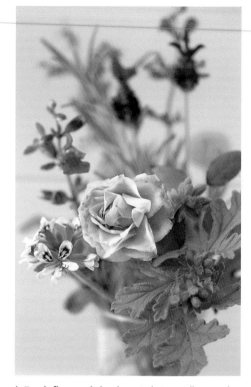

△ **Fresh flowers bring beauty into our lives and stimulate feelings of happiness and well-being.**

more popular essential oils, in general use, at this time. By the fifth month of pregnancy, the baby should be firmly attached to the uterus, and any essential oils can be used. All essential oils should be used only in the recommended dosage.

Some essential oils have components in them which may induce a period or which can affect the nervous system if overused. Some of these oils may help to stimulate the uterus into action, and they should be used only when labour commences, to relieve labour pains. Used correctly, essential oils can alleviate many of the minor discomforts of pregnancy. Many women also find them invaluable during labour to ease pain and to facilitate delivery. However, some controversy exists surrounding the use of some essential oils during pregnancy.

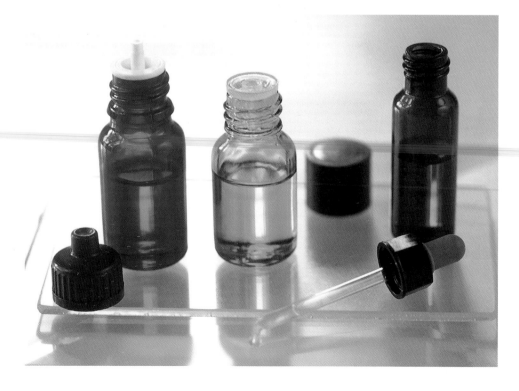

◁ **Two essential oils can be mixed together in an easy-to-use dropper bottle for effective self-treatment at home.**

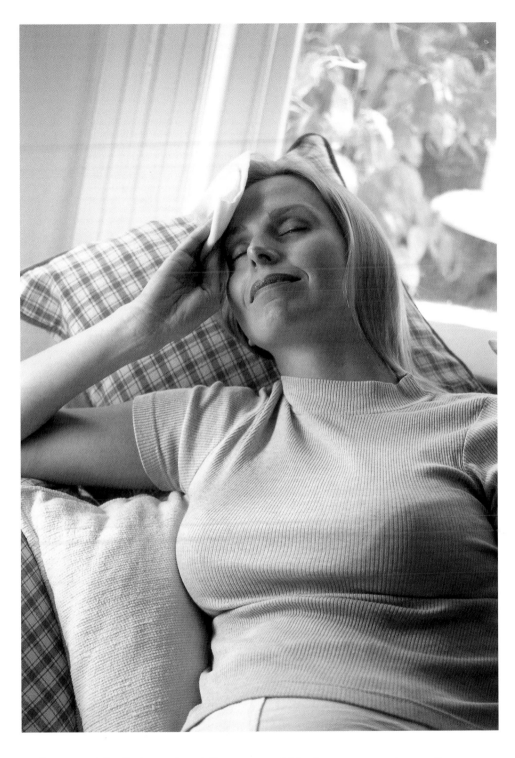

◁ A cool lavender compress can ease a tension headache. Lie or sit quietly in a place where you won't be disturbed and apply the compress to your temples or forehead until relief is felt.

▽ Whether this is your first pregnancy or whether you are already a mother, preparing for a new baby is an exciting time for all the family.

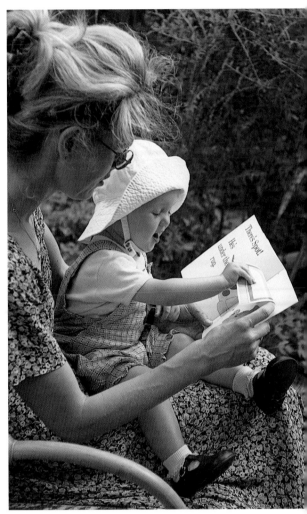

A few essential oils have the ability to stimulate uterine contractions, and could possibly cause miscarriage if taken in excessive amounts or taken internally during the first three to four months of pregnancy. Other oils can have an effect on the nervous system and the liver, and could be toxic when taken in too high a dose.

When oils are used correctly, the risks are very slight because of the low dosage involved (generally, five to ten drops at any one time). Women who have a history of miscarriage may be most at risk but, in any case, it is always better to err on the side of safety. Use only those essential oils which do not appear in any literature as being hazardous during pregnancy. There are many oils which will do you no harm at all but, if you are in any doubt about using an essential oil while pregnant, you should consult a qualified aromatherapist.

Whether pregnant or trying to start a family, the important thing to remember is that anything taken into the body, whether it is food, drink, nicotine, alcohol, or any other substance, will have an effect upon the system. Sensible eating with plenty of sleep and regular exercise is the best way to look after yourself and prepare your body and mind for motherhood.

OILS TO AVOID DURING THE FIRST HALF OF PREGNANCY

Although all essential oils are safe when used with care and knowledge, it is advised that you avoid the following oils, which can promote menstruation:

• aniseed *Pimpinella anisum*

• fennel *Foeniculum vulgare*

• nutmeg *Myristica fragrans*

• sage *Salvia officinalis*

• yarrow *Achillea millefolium*

In addition, avoid any essential oil that is new to you at this time.

Using aromatherapy in pregnancy

Essential oils can bring relief from the many minor troubles which can occur during pregnancy. Discomforts commonly experienced by women include morning sickness, backache, oedema (swollen legs and ankles), constipation, varicose veins, digestive problems (including heartburn), leg cramps and exhaustion. Coping with these discomforts can be especially difficult while the woman is working or if there is a small child or children to look after in the home. Essential oils are also useful during labour, to ease pain and to facilitate delivery.

morning sickness

Nausea, which typically occurs in the morning, is often one of the first signs that a woman is pregnant. Inhalations with a vaporizer can be helpful at bedtime and first thing in the morning. The oils can be left to vaporize overnight in the bedroom. If the sickness persists through the day, prepare a tissue with the relevant oils, and keep it with you at all times.

constipation

This is also another early sign of pregnancy. Prepare essential oils in a suitable carrier base and apply them to the abdomen in a

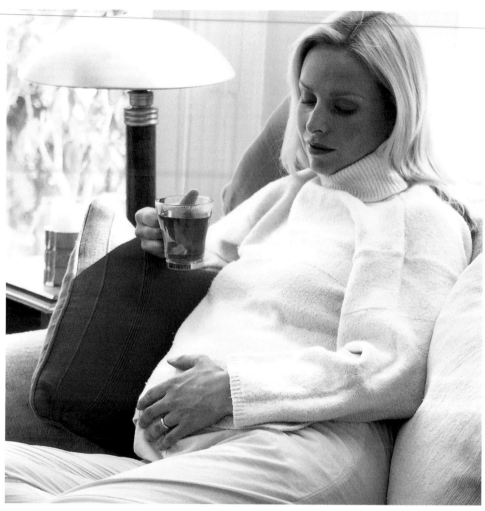

△ As your pregnancy proceeds, you will feel your baby's first movements. Setting aside some time each day to relax and be with your unborn child can help the mother-child bonding process.

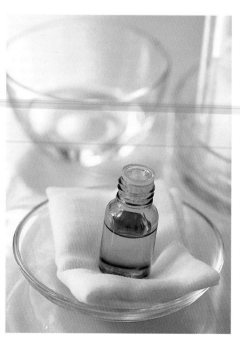

◁ Add a few drops of bitter orange to a bowl of water and make a compress to ease constipation.

clockwise direction. Alternatively, use the oils in the bath and/or on a compress. Eating a healthy diet and drinking plenty of water will help to reduce the risk of constipation.

stretch marks

By the beginning of the second trimester, your clothes will be feeling tighter as your abdomen swells. Halfway through this trimester you will be able to feel the baby's first movements (an exciting moment). Start using essential oils at this time to prevent stretch marks on the skin of the abdomen. Through the correct and diligent

application of appropriate essential oils it is possible to maintain a supple and undamaged skin, and you will greatly appreciate your efforts after the baby is born.

Prepare a carrier base (include calendula oil) containing oils with regenerative and skin-toning properties. The mixture should be applied to the abdomen twice daily, morning and night. The area to be covered increases as the pregnancy proceeds, and will include the sides of the body, the groin and on and above the breasts.

backache

As your baby grows, so the likelihood of backache increases. Sitting and standing with correct posture can go a long way to minimize backache, but it will usually occur at some stage and can be helped with essential oils when it does. Prepare a carrier base, then add the appropriate oils and ask a friend or your partner to give you a back massage, ideally at bedtime. Try using the same essential oils (but without the carrier oil) in the bath. Include basil and marjoram in the massage-mix; these can also be used if you suffer from leg cramps later on.

heartburn

The growing baby may also put pressure on your stomach, causing indigestion and heartburn. For heartburn, add 2 drops each of mandarin and peppermint oils to 10 ml (2 tsp) carrier base and apply to the painful area. These oils can also be inhaled neat from a tissue or cupped hands, breathing deeply.

varicose veins, swollen legs and ankles

It is as well for all women to watch out for early signs of these conditions through-out pregnancy. Resting with the feet and legs raised is beneficial for all leg conditions. Although the essential oils are different for each condition, the method of use is the same. Prepare a carrier base and add the oils.

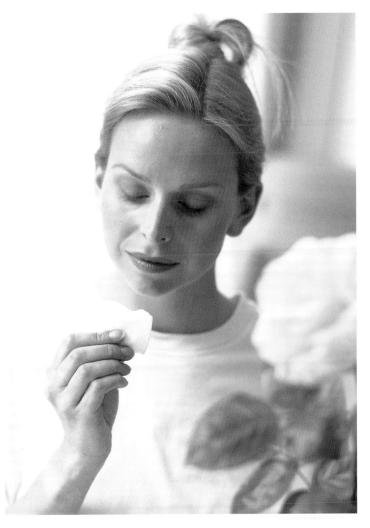

the reproductive years

◁ Your growing baby can cause painful heartburn. Put two drops each of mandarin and peppermint on a tissue and sniff throughout the day.

▽ Backache is a common complaint of pregnancy. Ask your partner for a back massage, using basil and marjoram, before going to bed.

Apply the mixture to the whole leg, then bring your hands firmly from the foot up to the knee, before returning to the foot to start again. Massage only in an upward direction, to encourage blood flow to the heart. For varicose veins on the upper leg, massage upwards, going only from knee to groin – not back again – several times.

◁ A room vaporizer is a convenient way of inhaling oils. To help with morning sickness, vaporize a combination of lemon, ginger and basil at bedtime and when you wake up.

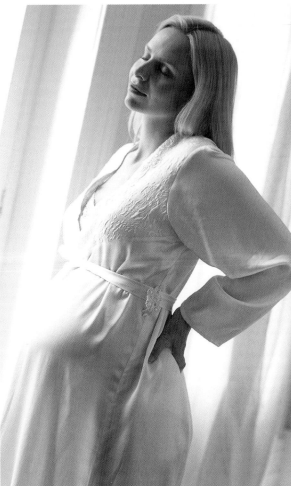

Ante-natal bodycare

During the last trimester of pregnancy, it is a good idea to prepare for labour and to discuss with your midwife or doctor how you would like the birth to proceed. It is helpful to attend prenatal classes, especially if it is the birth of your first child. The classes teach useful exercises to help you relax when the time for labour comes.

preparing for labour

Much of the pain of childbirth, particularly with a first child, is due to the muscles at the neck of the uterus and the perineum being tense and/or inflexible, which means they can tear when stretched. This can be eased by the application of muscle-relaxing essential oils in a vegetable carrier oil. If application is begun daily from several weeks before the expected birth date, the area can be made supple and soft. This will prepare it for the enormous amount of expansion needed for the baby to be born.

Massage a little of the mix twice daily around the perineum area, and try inserting your fingers into the neck of the womb to stretch it, thus helping to prevent tearing.

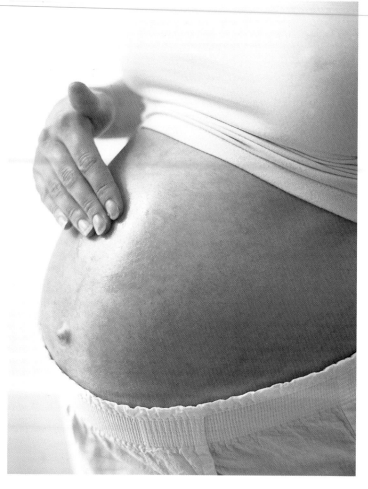

◁ **To prevent stretch marks, geranium and frankincense, in a calendula oil carrier, should be massaged on to the abdomen area twice daily.**

▽ **Massage the lower leg in an upwards direction to relieve aches and oedema.**

As you get heavier, remember to keep increasing the area to which you are applying your essential oil blend to prevent stretch marks, taking your mix round the sides of your body, on to the upper part of your thighs and above your breasts. It is also important at this time to rest your legs at regular intervals (from every five minutes to half an hour, if you suspect you are likely to develop varicose veins).

As the time for the birth approaches, you may experience conflicting emotions and mood swings. Using uplifting essential oils can give you inner strength to cope with all that is in store for you during this very exciting time in your life.

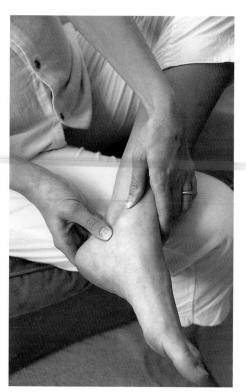

◁ **Make regular checks for oedema on your feet and ankles as your pregnancy progresses. If symptoms occur, a massage plan can help.**

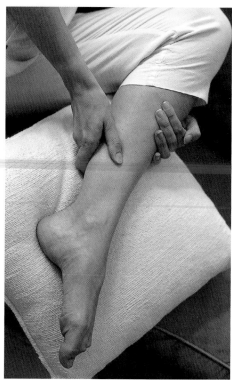

Relief treatments for labour

There are some oils which are particularly useful in labour. In the past, these were limited to lavender and clary sage for their calming and relaxing effects. However, there are a few oils with womb-stimulant and analgesic properties, and these can help with contractions: aniseed, clove bud, nutmeg and sage. These oils are *absolutely not* advocated for the first four months of pregnancy and should not be used until the last week, when labour is about to begin. Used correctly, these oils can help to make the birth easier and quicker, especially for a first-time mother. They are used to relieve pain and induce sleep, and will have a soothing, dulling, lulling effect. Clove bud is particularly analgesic and nutmeg is an effective sedative.

treatment

Try a mix of two drops each of any two of the oils with four drops of lavender on a tissue, and inhale between contractions. Some women like to put the tissue into the switched-off gas and air machine, which seems to have the psychological effect of making the oils more efficient.

Alternatively, blend three drops each of aniseed, nutmeg and peppermint with eight drops of lavender into 50 ml (2 fl oz) carrier oil, and ask your partner to massage your feet and lower legs every half hour. Apply the same mix to your own hands and shoulders, if preferred.

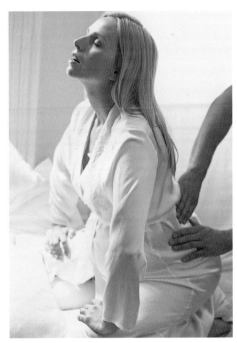

▷ **Lower back pain can be eased by massage. Ask your partner to rub the painful areas.**

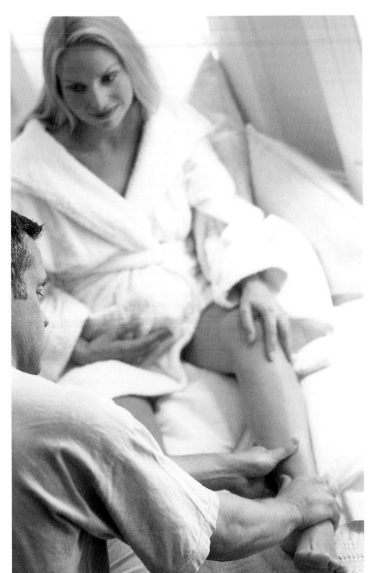

◁ **Peppermint and aniseed are analgesic and antispasmodic. Combined with lavender, a blend can be massaged on to the lower legs during labour to ease pain.**

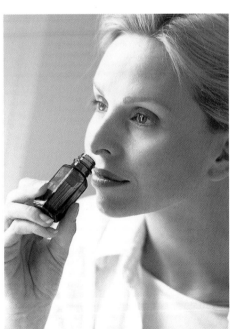

▷ **Inhalation is the fastest method for an oil's aroma to reach the brain. Aniseed and lavender are calming and can help with contractions.**

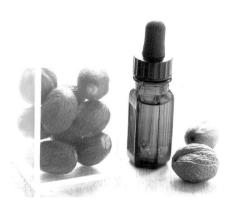

▷ **Nutmeg is a very useful oil for the last stages of labour as it relieves pain and can facilitate delivery. Consult a qualified aromatherapist if you wish to use it.**

Post-natal bodycare

Essential oils can be used to help with the common emotional stresses and physical problems arising as a result of the birth.

Use 6 drops of the appropriate essential oils blended in 20 ml (4 tsp) of calendula oil for application. Alternatively, use them on their own for inhalation or in the bath.

birth wounds

During the birth, the perineum may be bruised and/or torn, and can be very painful afterwards. Using the three perineum oils, gently apply them several times a day. If the area is too painful to touch, use a compress (see Aromatherapy Techniques).

breast feeding problems

Always apply the appropriate essential oils immediately after each feed, so that they are completely absorbed by your body before the baby's next feed is due.

Insufficient milk: fennel oil encourages milk production. Fennel will also help to keep the baby's excreta normal and can help to relieve any wind.

Too much milk: 2 drops of peppermint oil with 4 drops of geranium oil can be used in a massage all over the breasts.

Cracked nipples or mastitis: use 2 drops of each essential oil listed opposite.

emotional difficulties

After the birth, it will take a while before your hormones return to normal. This can be a stressful time as you have a new baby to care for just when you are feeling in need of care yourself. Fatigue, anxiety, despondency and emotional imbalances are common. Essential oils can help before post-natal depression sets in. Blend oils for use by inhalation, in the bath or by application.

treating your baby

Essential oils can help you and your baby cope with the everyday, minor ailments which many babies are subject to, such as

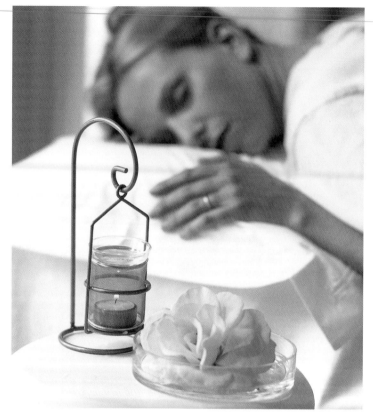

◁ **After a long and exhausting labour, and with a new baby to look after, make sure you get enough sleep. Burn lavender through the night to relax and refresh you.**

▽ **Once your baby is born, pamper yourself and invest in some good quality skincare products.**

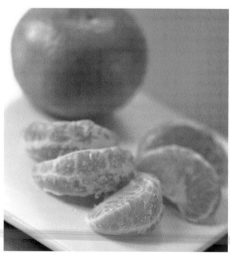

△ **The gentle action of mandarin makes it a good choice for treating colic and digestive disorders.**

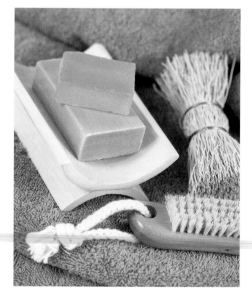

indigestion, colic, constipation and/or diarrhoea, minor infections and nappy rash. For nappy rash, use 15 ml (3 tsp) base lotion with 5 ml (1 tsp) calendula oil, mixed with one drop of peppermint and up to three drops of any other selected oils.

Babies can benefit from massage with essential oils. The massage will relax them

and can help to strengthen the bond between mother and child. For application to babies, use one drop of essential oil per 5 ml (1 tsp) carrier lotion or oil. For sleep problems, try two to three drops of oil in a vaporizer in the baby's room, or try them on a tissue which is pinned to the baby's clothes or placed inside the pillowcase.

Useful essential oils

essential oil	treatment
hormone-like essential oils	
Chamomile (German) *Matricaria recutica*	hormone-like
Clary sage *Salvia sclarea*	oestrogen-like
Niaouli *Melaleuca viridiflora*	oestrogen-like (regularizes periods)
backache	
Basil *Ocimum basilicum* var. *album*	analgesic, antispasmodic
Lavender *Lavandula angustifolia*	analgesic, anti-inflammatory, antispasmodic
Marjoram (sweet) *Origanum majorana*	analgesic, antispasmodic
constipation	
Ginger *Zingiber officinale*	analgesic, digestive stimulant
Mandarin *Citrus reticulata*	antispasmodic, calming, digestive stimulant
Orange (bitter) *Citrus aurantium* var. *amara*	calming, digestive stimulant
Rosemary *Rosmarinus officinalis*	analgesic, digestive stimulant
nausea	
Basil *Ocimum basilicum* var. *album*	digestive tonic, nervous system regulator
Ginger *Zingiber officinale*	digestive
Lemon *Citrus limon*	anticoagulant, antispasmodic, calming, digestive
stretch marks	
Frankincense *Boswellia carteri*	cell regenerative, cicatrizant (scars)
Geranium *Pelargonium graveolens*	cell regenerative, cicatrizant (stretch marks)
Lavender *Lavandula angustifolia*	cicatrizant (scars)
fluid retention	
Fennel *Foeniculum vulgare*	diuretic (cellulite, oedema)
Juniper *Juniperus communis*	diuretic (cellulite, oedema)
Lemon *Citrus limon*	diuretic (obesity, oedema)
varicose veins	
Clary sage *Salvia sclarea*	phlebotonic (circulatory problems, haemorrhoids, varicose veins)
Cypress *Cupressus sempervirens*	phlebotonic (haemorrhoids, poor venous circulation, varicose veins)
Niaouli *Melaleuca viridiflora*	phlebotonic (haemorrhoids, varicose veins)

essential oil	treatment
labour	
Aniseed *Pimpinella anisum*	analgesic, antispasmodic, calming (gentle narcotic), emmenagogic, oestrogen-like, uterotonic
Lavender *Lavandula angustifolia*	analgesic, antispasmodic, calming (anxiety), sedative
Nutmeg *Myristica fragrans*	analgesic, sedative (narcotic), neurotonic, uterotonic
Peppermint *Mentha* x *piperita*	analgesic, antispasmodic, hormone-like (ovarian stimulant), neurotonic, uterotonic (facilitates delivery)
perineum	
Geranium *Pelargonium graveolens*	analgesic, cicatrizant (wounds)
Lavender *Lavandula angustifolia*	analgesic, antiseptic (bruises)
Rosemary *Rosmarinus officinalis*	analgesic, anti-inflammatory
breast milk	
Fennel *Foeniculum vulgare*	lactogenic (promotes milk), oestrogen-like (insufficient milk)
Geranium *Pelargonium graveolens*	decongestant (breast congestion – for too much milk)
Peppermint *Mentha* x *piperita*	antilactogenic (prevents milk forming)
cracked nipples or mastitis	
Chamomile (German) *Matricaria recutica*	cicatrizant (infected wounds, ulcers)
Geranium *Pelargonium graveolens*	cicatrizant (burns, cuts, ulcers, wounds)
Lavender *Lavandula angustifolia*	cicatrizant (burns, scars, varicose veins, wounds)
nappy rash	
Patchouli *Pogostemon patchouli*	anti-inflammatory, cicatrizant (cracked skin, scar tissue)
Peppermint *Mentha* x *piperita*	analgesic, anti-inflammatory, soothing (skin irritation, rashes)
post-natal depression	
Basil *Ocimum basilicum* var. *album*	nervous system regulator (anxiety), neurotonic (convalescence, depression)
Chamomile (Roman) *Chamaemelum nobile*	calming (nervous depression, nervous shock)

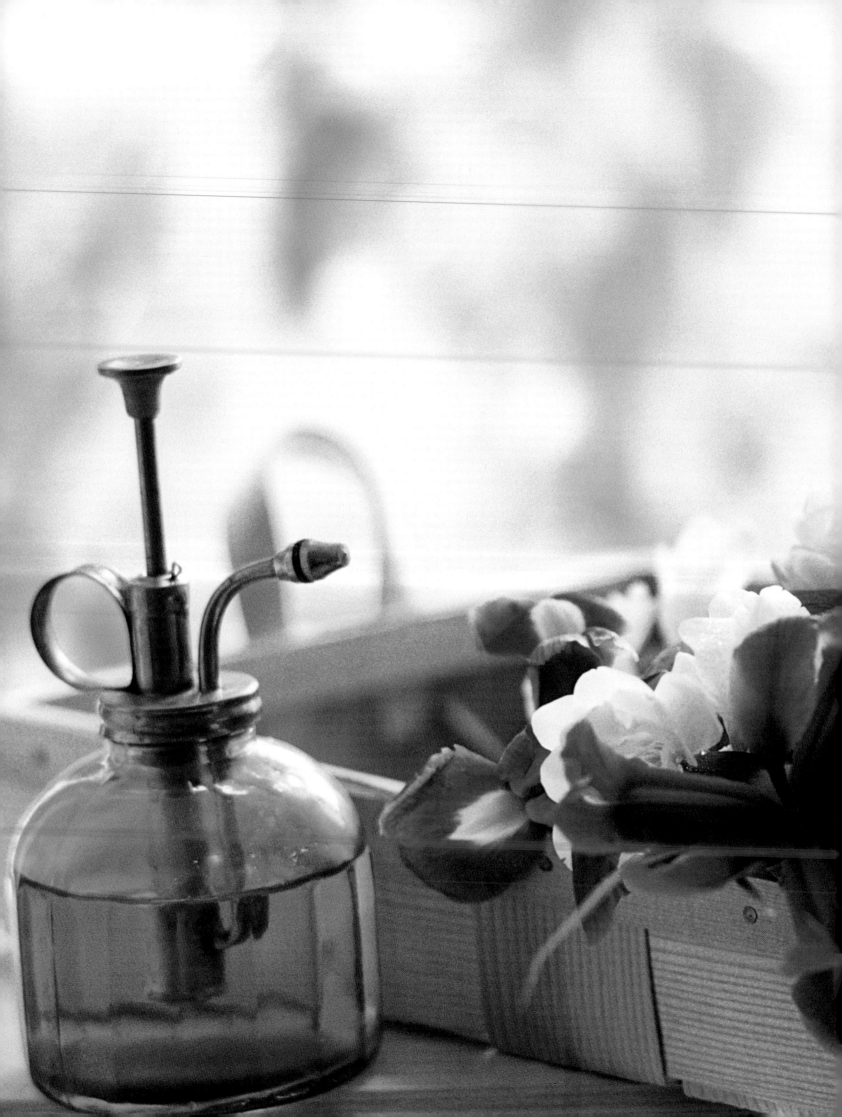

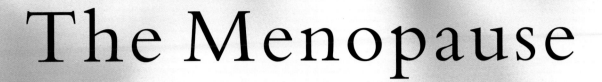

The Menopause

Softly on the evening hour,

Secret herbs their spices shower,

Dark-spiked rosemary and myrrh,

Lean-stalked purple lavender.

From The Sunken Garden, Walter de la Mare, 1873–1956.

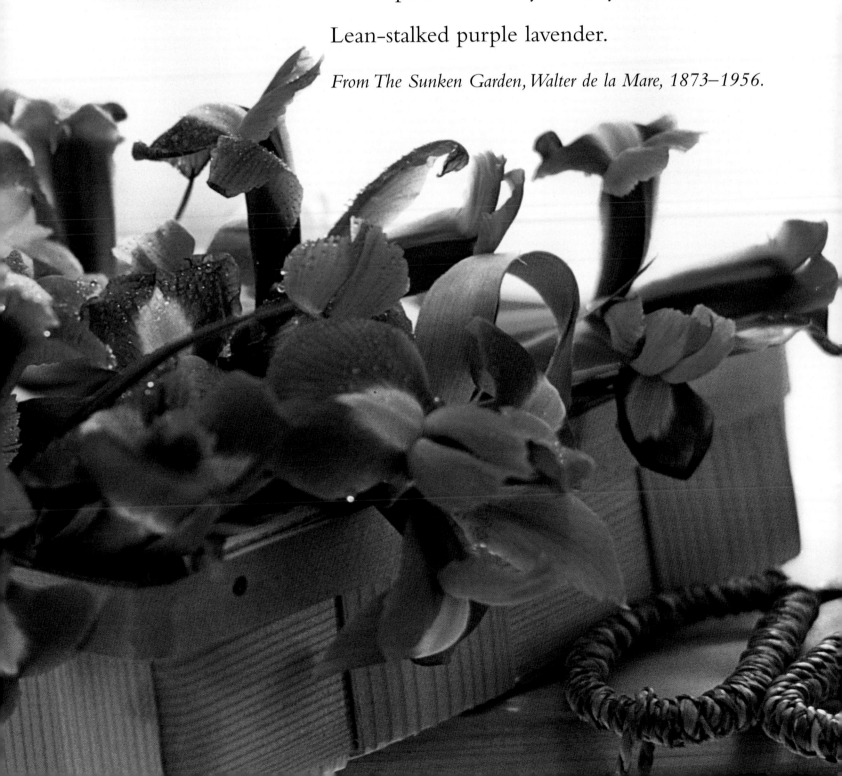

The menopause

The word menopause derives from the Greek words for month, *men*, and halt, *pausis*. It refers to the end of menstruation, when a woman's ovaries no longer produce eggs for fertilization and her periods stop. The accepted average age at which the menopause occurs is 51, with around five per cent of women ceasing their periods before they are 45.

The menopause does not happen overnight. It is a gradual process brought about by growing irregularity in, and gradual reduction of, the reproductive hormones, oestrogen and progesterone. Oestrogen is probably the most important hormone concerned with a woman's health: it helps to lower cholesterol levels, protect against heart attacks and strokes, to preserve bone tissue and regulate mood and behaviour patterns. Instability occurs in the mental and physical body because of these reduced hormone levels. The early stages of the menopause can present similar emotional imbalances to PMS, and physical symptoms, to varying degrees of severity, may also develop.

As with menstruation, different women will be affected in different ways by the menopause. For women who have had a lifetime of period-associated problems, the menopause may come as a welcome relief.

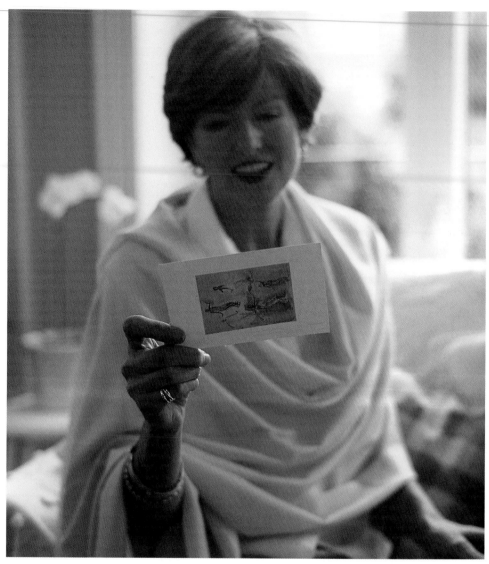

△ **The menopause is a major life transition. How we cope with it will depend to some extent on our mental attitude. Staying in touch with friends and leading an active life can help us to feel positive.**

She is clothed with strength and dignity and can laugh at years to come. She speaks with wisdom and faithful instruction is on her tongue.

From Proverbs 31:25 The Holy Bible.

Once a woman's periods have stopped for a year, there is no longer any need to worry about becoming pregnant or, therefore, to practise any form of birth control. Some women experience few or no problems at all with the menopause, yet for others, this can be a difficult time as their bodies adjust to a major life change.

Other physical changes may be noticed, affecting the skin and hair, the activity of the thyroid glands and the distribution of body fat. Some women may experience sudden haemorrhaging, headaches, dizzy spells and sleep disturbances.

osteoporosis

One of the more serious potential side effects of the menopause is the development of osteoporosis, which is caused by lack of oestrogen production. This is when the bones of the body become increasingly fragile and brittle. The bones fracture easily, particularly at the more vulnerable points such as the wrists, ankles or hip joints in the event of physical stress, such as a fall. Osteoporosis is also responsible for the eventual development of stooping shoulders in older women, often referred to as a "dowager's hump".

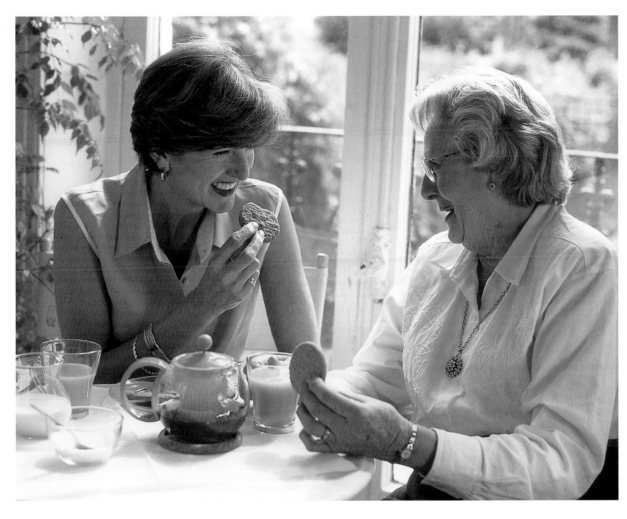

◁ **With the children grown up, you are likely to have more time for yourself. Now is a good time to catch up with family and friends.**

Hormone replacement therapy

Advances in medical science now mean that synthetic hormone replacements can offset the symptoms of the menopause. Many women decide to try hormone replacement therapy (HRT) if they find that the discomforts of the menopause are affecting their quality of life. HRT is not suitable for all women, however, and much will depend on the needs and medical background of the individual. Because HRT is still a relatively new treatment, its long-term effects are not yet fully known. Treatments are now available from your doctor which are made with natural progesterone. These are believed to be safer than treatments using synthetic oestrogen, and this will make them popular with many women.

Some menopausal symptoms can also be helped by aromatherapy. Clary sage is one of several oestrogen-like essential oils. It is worth using essential oils on a regular basis to see how your symptoms are affected before deciding on HRT.

▽ **Clary sage and cypress can help with night sweats. Prepare a mix and use it at bedtime.**

COMMON SYMPTOMS OF THE MENOPAUSE
- Hot flushes
- Night sweats
- Depression
- Sweating
- Fatigue
- Water retention
- Vaginal dryness

▷ **Some women choose to spend more time on gardening or other hobbies, while others may decide to retrain and embark on a new career.**

Common symptoms of menopause

Although a large percentage of women have no problems with the menopause, many do experience some discomfort.

night sweats

These are best tackled through preventative treatment. Try taking an aromatherapy bath with the relevant oils each night before bedtime. Alternatively, try massaging the oils in a suitable carrier base into the body.

hot flushes

Put 20 drops of the same blend of essential oils in 1 litre (1¾ pints) of spring water in a screw-topped bottle. Fit the lid, shake well and transfer some into a purse-size spray and some into a small bottle that you can carry around with you. As soon as you feel a flush coming on, drink two mouthfuls of the water and spray your face and neck. Vitamin E is also said to be effective.

water retention and bloating

To reduce water retention and cellulite, the relevant essential oils should be added to a suitable carrier base and applied daily to the affected areas. The same oils can also be used neat in the bath.

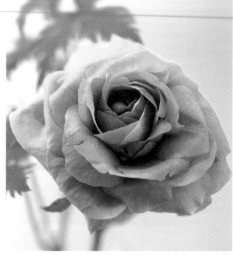

△ **Rose otto can help with haemorrhaging. It is also useful for both loss of libido and dry skin.**

hair and skin

The condition of the hair and skin can be affected by the hormonal changes of the menopause. Both will become thinner and drier, and it is a good idea to adapt your daily care regime to compensate.

hair

For hair dryness, use a good conditioner. You may like to add appropriate essential oils to give extra shine. For thinning hair, try a daily scalp massage with essential oils (*see* Aromatherapy Techniques).

skin

This not only becomes drier, but is more prone to wrinkles. Try a product containing essential oils or prepare your own mix.

haemorrhaging

Occasional and sudden bleeding can occur when you least expect it. Although essential oils can reduce the amount of blood loss, as far as we know, they do not seem to stop it happening. As a preventative measure, try using styptic and/or astringent essential oils if you are prone to haemorrhaging.

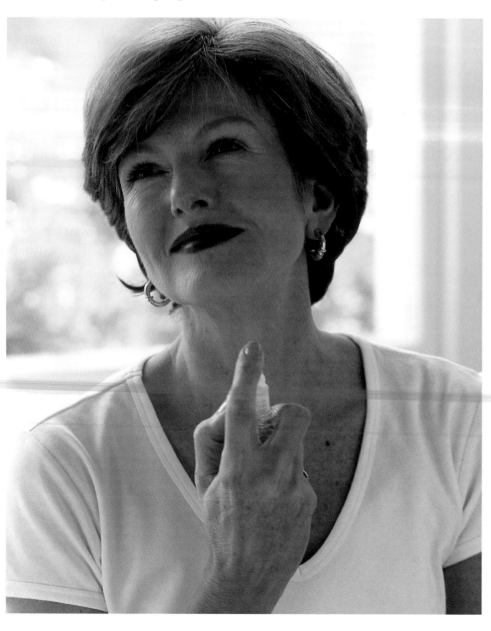

◁ **Peppermint and cypress are useful for hot flushes. Make up a mix and use it in an atomizer.**

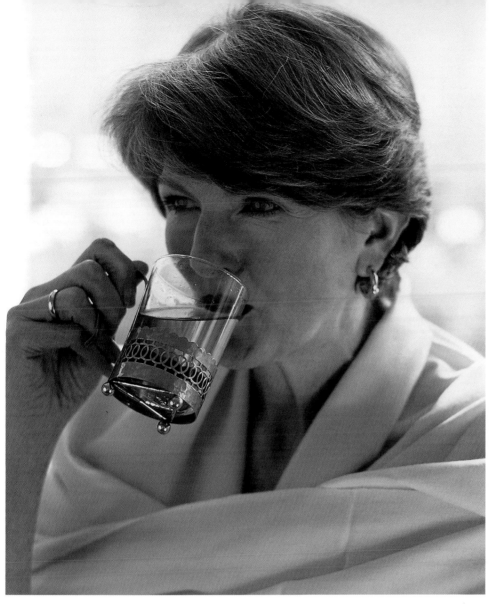

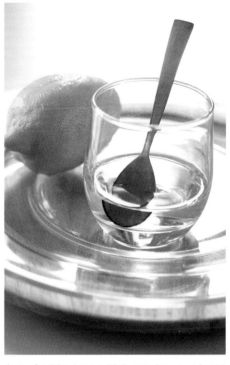

△ A refreshing lemon drink can give you a boost and relieve depression. As always, special care should be taken with oils for internal use.

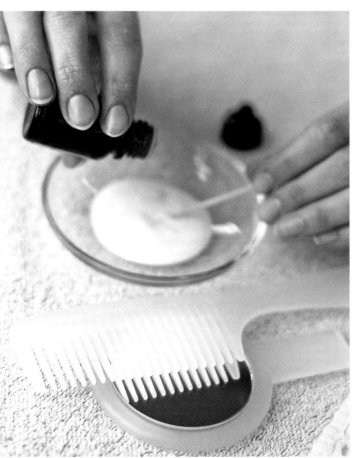

△ If you are having difficulties sleeping, a soothing cup of sweet marjoram and chamomile tea in the evening can help.

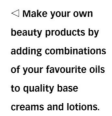

◁ Make your own beauty products by adding combinations of your favourite oils to quality base creams and lotions.

heart and circulation problems

In developed countries, arterial disease is the commonest cause of death for women over 50, killing one in four. This is almost twice as high as the death-rate from cancer.

There are as yet no essential oils known to treat problems with the heart, and it is advisable to check with your doctor and your family history to see if you are at risk. In the meantime, you can help to prevent heart and blood-pressure problems by giving up smoking, avoiding fatty foods and drinks high in caffeine, eating a low-cholesterol diet and taking enough regular exercise. There are also some carrier oils reputed to reduce cholesterol levels.

vaginal dryness

This can cause both emotional and physical discomfort. There are no known essential oils to increase vaginal fluid. Vitamin E is reputed to improve vaginal secretion, and daily application of sunflower oil all round the vaginal opening may also help.

Emotions during menopause

For many women the menopause will coincide with their children leaving home. It can represent a new lease of life as a woman suddenly finds that she has more time for herself. However, as with any major life change, the menopause is often accompanied by mixed feelings, and a woman's new-found freedom may be marred not only by physical symptoms but also by emotional disturbances.

stress-related headaches and sleep disturbances

These disturbances are not necessarily linked to the menopause, and may be stress-related. However, should either of them bother you, inhalation and application of the appropriate essential oils can help.

weight and diet

Appearance is often important to a woman throughout her life. It is not surprising, then, that poor self-esteem and a lack of confidence can be triggered by the physical changes happening in her body at this time.

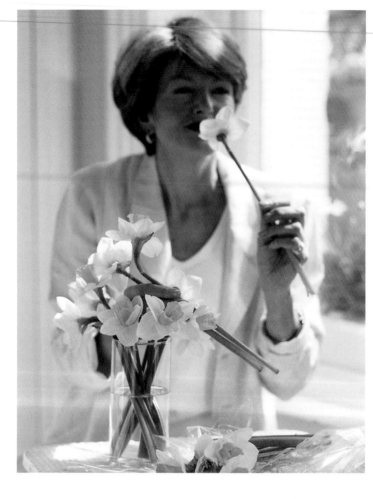

◁ **During the menopause, you may experience strong mood swings. Try to keep things in proportion and take pleasure from the simple things in life.**

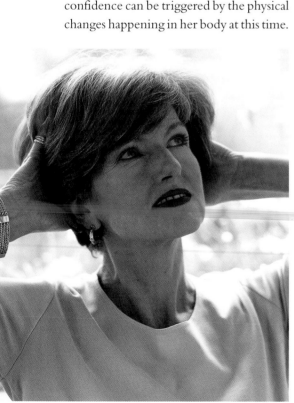

△ **When you are feeling tired and irritable, a head massage can help you to relax and unwind.**

Water retention can lead to bloating and weight-gain which, in turn, will exacerbate any feelings of low self-esteem. Tackle this with a positive frame of mind and healthy eating habits – these two things combined will improve self-confidence. Essential oils used for low spirits may help weight loss by stimulating the nervous system.

EMOTIONAL DISTURBANCES OF THE MENOPAUSE

• Irritability

• Lack of confidence

• Anxiety and depression

• Poor concentration, forgetfulness and memory problems

• Decrease in self-esteem: through weight gain, lack of interest in sex, changes in physical appearance

tips for healthy eating and drinking

• Drink plenty of water.

• Limit alcohol intake to two units a day.

• Cut down on caffeine drinks.

• Cut down on, or avoid, sugary foods and foods high in fat.

• Eat more fish and less meat (especially red meat); eat plenty of fruit and vegetables, especially those rich in Vitamin C.

• Include foods rich in calcium.

loss of sex drive

For some women, the menopause is marked by a decrease in sex drive (conversely, some women also report an increase in libido). The reduction in vaginal fluid can make intercourse painful, and this can lead to a change in sexual desire.

Several essential oils are reputed to help with sexual problems and to increase desire. These oils relax the mind, relieving it from pressures and tensions and, at the same time, can stimulate the emotions. Use the appropriate oils in a vaporizer for an hour before retiring, in both the living room and the bedroom. Alternatively, sprinkle a few drops of the oils on to your pillow and exchange a gentle back and shoulder aromatherapy massage with your partner.

relationship difficulties

The physical and emotional difficulties of the menopause can put a strain on your relationship with your partner. If your children are leaving home, now may be a good time to re-define your partnership. It can help to blend stress-relieving essential oils with oils which correspond to your emotions, such as anger, fear or jealousy.

▷ **Emotional upsets are stressful and can lead to muscular tension. Rub oils on to your shoulders and neck to help restore your equilibrium.**

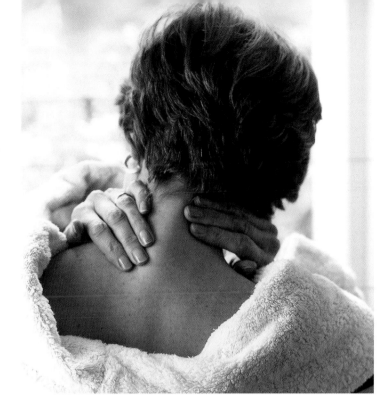

Useful essential oils

essential oil	treatment
hot flushes and sweating	
Clary sage *Salvia sclarea*	antisudorific, oestrogen-like (sweating)
Cypress *Cupressus sempervirens*	antisudorific (excessive perspiration)
Peppermint *Mentha x piperita*	cooling
Pine *Pinus sylvestris*	antisudorific (sweating)
reputed sexual stimulants	
Peppermint *Mentha x piperita*	neurotonic, reproductive tonic
Rosemary *Rosmarinus officinalis*	neurotonic, sexual tonic
Rose otto *Rosa damascena*	neurotonic, sexual tonic
Thyme (sweet) *Thymus vulgaris*	cardiotonic, immunostimulant, neurotonic, sexual tonic
Ylang ylang *Cananga odorata*	reproductive tonic
low spirits (depression) and fatigue	
Basil *Ocimum basilicum* var. *album*	neurotonic debility, mental strain, depression
Chamomile (Roman) *Chamaemelum nobile*	calming (nervous depression, irritability, nervous shock)
Clary sage *Salvia sclarea*	neurotonic (nervous fatigue)
Cypress *Cupressus sempervirens*	neurotonic (debility)
Frankincense *Boswellia carteri*	antidepressive (nervous depression)
Geranium *Pelargonium graveolens*	neurotonic (debility, nervous fatigue)
Juniper *Juniperus communis*	neurotonic (debility, fatigue)
Marjoram (sweet) *Origanum majorana*	neurotonic (debility, anguish, agitation, nervous depression)
Rosemary *Rosmarinus officinalis*	neurotonic (general debility and fatigue)

essential oil	treatment
fluid retention and cellulite	
Cypress *Cupressus sempervirens*	diuretic (oedema, rheumatic swelling)
Geranium *Pelargonium graveolens*	decongestant (lymphatic congestion)
headaches and sleep problems	
Chamomile (Roman) *Chamaemelum nobile*	antispasmodic, calming (migraines, insomnia, irritability)
Lavender *Lavandula angustifolia*	analgesic, calming (headaches, migraines, insomnia – low dose)
Marjoram (sweet) *Origanum majorana*	analgesic, calming (agitation, migraines, insomnia)
headaches and migraines only	
Peppermint *Mentha x piperita*	analgesic (headaches, migraine)
Rosemary *Rosmarinus officinalis*	decongestant (headaches, migraine)
irritability	
Chamomile (Roman) *Chamaemelum nobile*	calming (irritability, nervous depression, nervous shock)
Cypress *Cupressus sempervirens*	calming (irritability), regulates sympathetic nervous system
haemorrhage	
Cypress *Cupressus sempervirens*	astringent, phlebotonic (broken capillaries, varicose veins)
Rose otto *Rosa damascena*	astringent, styptic (wounds)

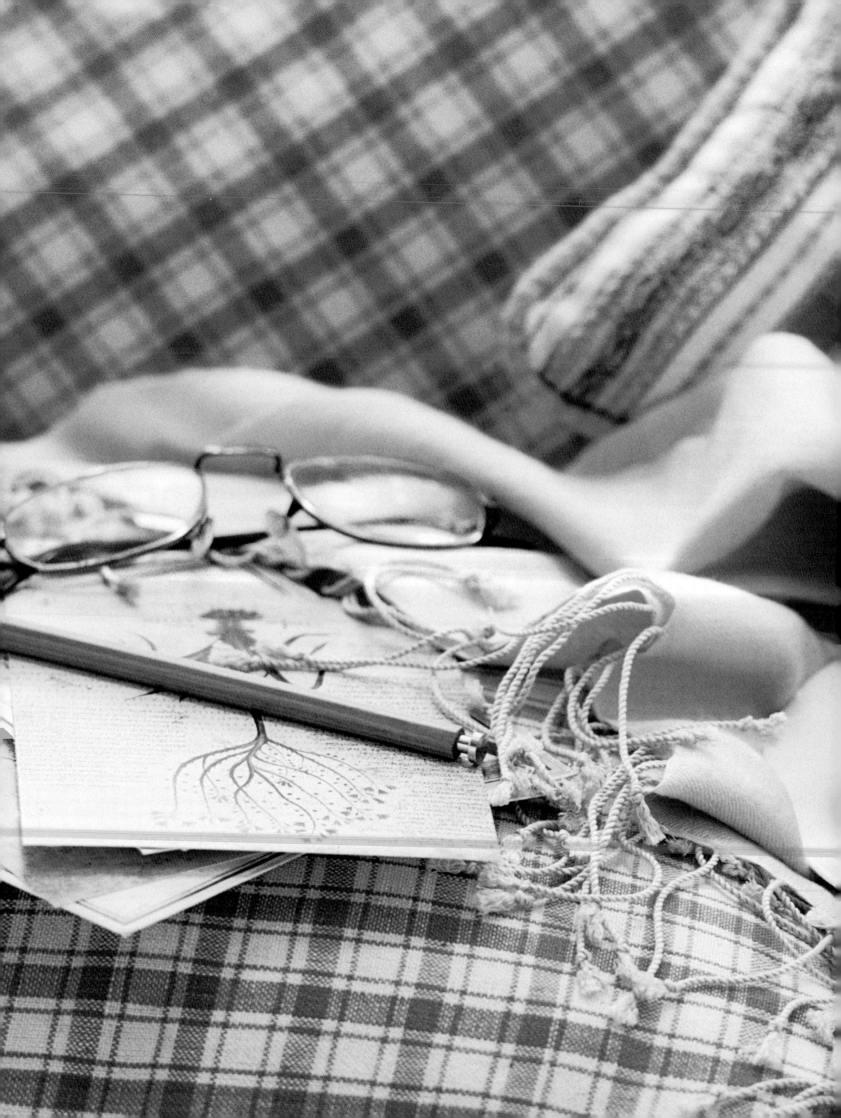

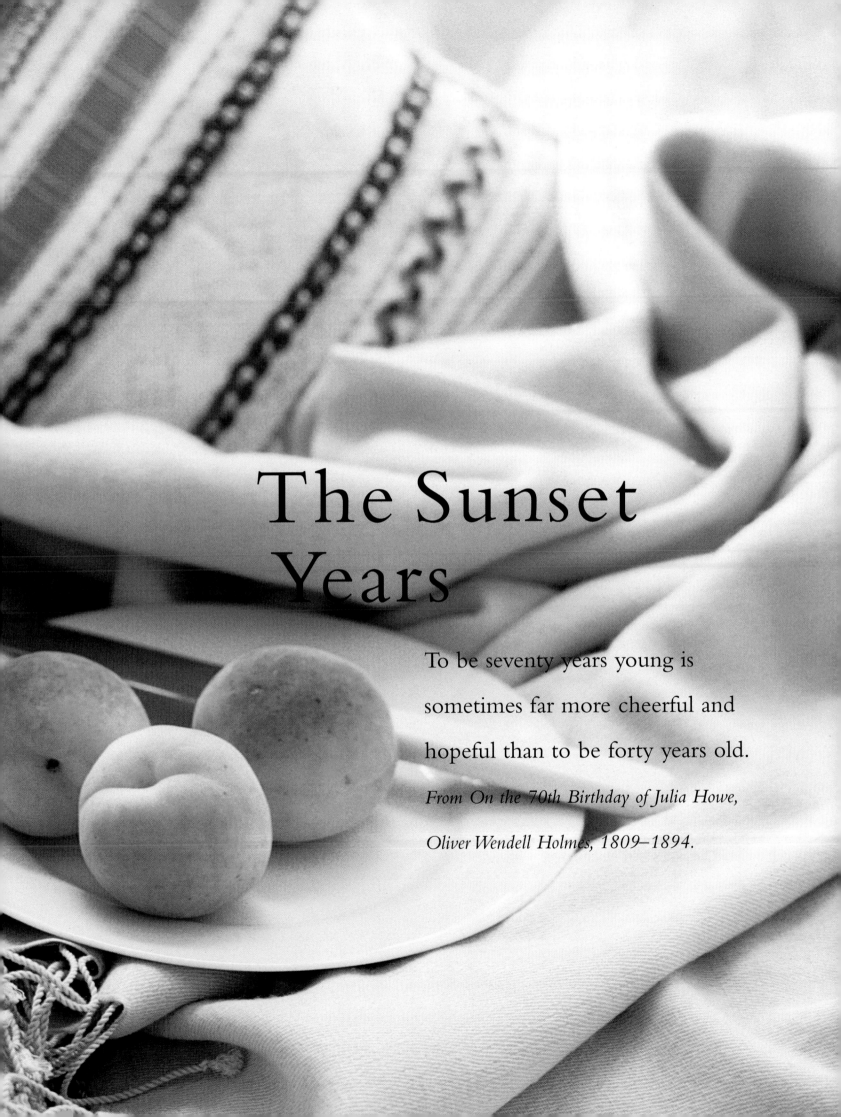

The Sunset Years

To be seventy years young is sometimes far more cheerful and hopeful than to be forty years old.

From On the 70th Birthday of Julia Howe,

Oliver Wendell Holmes, 1809–1894.

Aging gracefully

Once the menopause is over women enter a new phase of life, sometimes referred to as "the sunset years", before reaching old-age. During these years it is especially important for women to take care of themselves so as to prolong a happy, healthy and active life.

During the aging process, circulation slows down and the body's cells neither receive nourishment nor have harmful toxins eliminated as quickly as before. As a result, circulatory disorders are common: the hands and feet become cold, and wounds take longer to heal, for example. Digestive disorders in the elderly are also quite common. As the digestive processes slow down and the large intestine muscles weaken, constipation may occur. This is made more likely by inadequate roughage and fibre in the diet, and can also be seen as a side effect of other medicines. Eating while anxious or frightened can also bring on a variety of digestive disorders.

All cell renewal takes longer with age, the skin becomes dry and flaky, and the hair often becomes thinner. Because of this

> **An essence of balm (melissa) given in Canary wine every morning will renew youth, strengthen the brain, relieve languishing nature and prevent baldness.**
>
> *From the London Dispensary, 1696.*

slowing down process, every organ of every system in the body is more susceptible to common illnesses, which are more difficult to shake off. Older people are particularly vulnerable to colds and 'flu, which can settle on the chest, causing or exacerbating respiratory problems such as bronchitis and asthma. The joints gradually become less flexible and the muscles are more prone to inflammation, and conditions such as arthritis or rheumatism may develop or get worse. As it is often first highlighted during the menopause, osteoporosis can become a problem, with the skeletal bones becoming more brittle: falls resulting in broken bones, such as the hip, are much more common in later years.

For many women, the prospect of old age is very frightening and creates tension and anxiety. Many women worry about the possibility of incapacitating illnesses, such as dementia, Parkinson's or Alzheimer's disease. Others suffer frequent headaches, migraines, insomnia and digestive upsets, which may be caused by the side effects of medical drugs that are being taken for other conditions. In fact, the side effects of medication can be responsible for many ailments apparent in older people. This can set up a vicious circle, where new medicines are prescribed to deal with the side effects of the original drug and which, in turn, can eventually lead to even more unpleasant

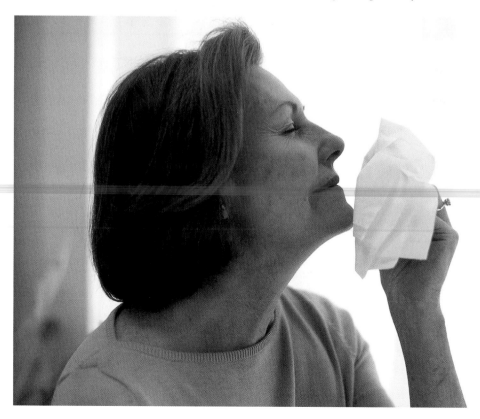

◁ **Extra care should be taken with a cold as it can develop into bronchitis. Use pine and niaouli on a tissue and inhale throughout the day.**

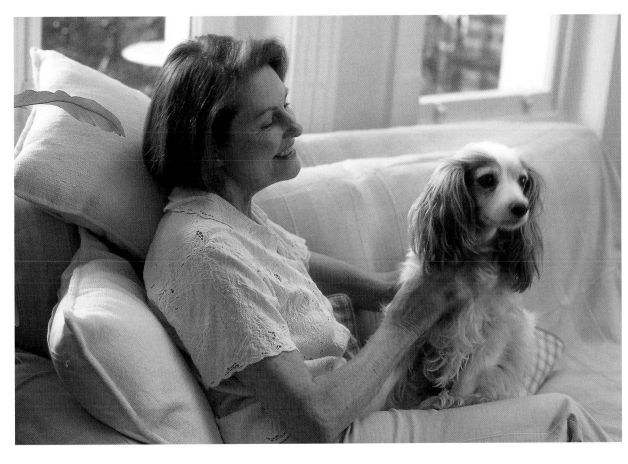

Striking a healthy balance between relaxation and activity is important. Besides keeping you company, a dog will encourage you to take a daily walk.

symptoms. These resulting afflictions are termed iatrogenic because they arise as the side effects of medication taken for the original disease or problem. Aromatherapy is now used in a growing number of hospitals to alleviate the more minor, but unpleasant, effects of iatrogenic disease: insomnia and digestive disorders are the most common, followed by pressure sores for those who are bedridden.

aromatherapy in later life

For women in their later years the amount of essential oils to be used in any treatment depends on the state of their general health. For those in good mental and physical health, the normal number of drops can be used. For women who are run down, suffering ill-health or are on medication the dosage should be lowered, as follows (*see also* Aromatherapy Techniques).

dosage

in the bath 4–6 drops of oil dispersed or dissolved first in dairy cream or honey
for application to the body 8–10 drops in 50 ml (3½ tbsp) carrier lotion
for inhalation the number of drops here is not crucial as many of the molecules are carried away by evaporation.

When preparing oils for application, a lotion is the preferred choice for a carrier base: oil bases can cause bottles to become too slippery and messy, often resulting in oil stains. If you suffer from arthritis, for example, you can add the relevant essential oils to a base hand and/or body lotion, to make the treatment easier to administer.

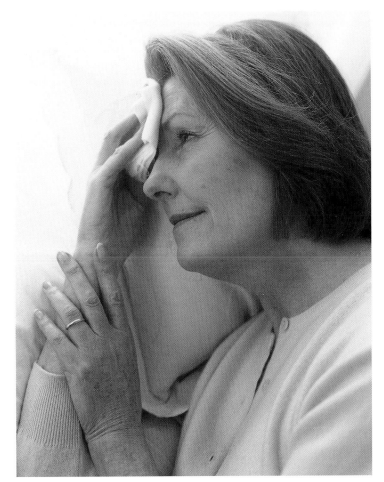

Holding a cotton pad with a few drops each of sweet marjoram and melissa to your head can relieve a tension headache. If it persists, try adding a few drops of Roman chamomile.

Strengthening physical health

In our sunset years, we have the time to look after our health. Now is the time to use essential oils as a safeguard against problems starting in the first place.

circulatory disorders

The regular daily use of hand and/or body lotion containing the appropriate essential oils will maintain a healthy circulation. Used early enough this could delay and, in some cases, prevent, many circulatory problems occurring.

After a stroke, the daily application of a lotion blend to legs and arms, in an upward direction only (to aid blood flow towards the heart), can help to regain movement in affected limbs.

varicose ulcers

These ulcers can originate from varicose veins, but they can also arise as secondary symptoms of diabetes, sickle-cell anaemia and rheumatoid arthritis. Essential oils dispersed in water and sprayed on to the area is the best method if the ulcers are too raw to touch. A compress is the next step, followed by application with oils in a calendula base as soon as the area can be touched.

arthritis, rheumatism and osteoarthritis

The main symptoms of arthritis are pain and stiffness, and of rheumatoid arthritis, inflammation and swelling around the joints, especially the knuckles, wrists, knees and ankles. Osteoarthritis is degeneration of the joint cartilage. A common site is the hip and, often, the only cure is to have an artificial hip replacement. Aromatherapy helps to alleviate pain and improve mobility in arthritic joints. The recommended treatment is the twice-daily use of a lotion containing relevant essential oils. SRT (*see* Swiss Reflex Therapy) is highly beneficial for arthritic hips and knees. Use overnight compresses for affected hands and feet.

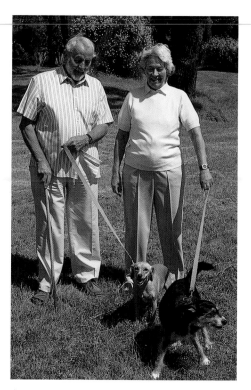

△ **Gentle exercise helps to keep arthritis at bay and maintain a healthy circulatory system.**

bronchial asthma and bronchitis

Many of the expectorant essential oils, which ease breathing, come from the conifer and melaleuca families, such as pine and niaouli. Try application of the oils in a carrier lotion, rubbed into the chest at bedtime. If a visit to hospital is necessary for any reason, take the lotion with you as it will help to prevent infections, such as pneumonia, which are often picked up in hospital. A daily foot massage using SRT (*see* Swiss Reflex Therapy) is also helpful.

influenza

Many essential oils are anti-infectious and can be of great help against influenza if they are used early enough: the sooner they are used after the onset of symptoms, the more likely they are to give a positive result. With the onset of a sore throat or fever, add the oils to water and use them as a gargle (*see* Aromatherapy Techniques). Try inhalations, aromatherapy baths, or direct application of the oils on to the body via a carrier lotion.

Preparing a multi-purpose treatment cream

It can be very useful to have a ready-mixed treatment to hand in case it is needed urgently. Choose an unperfumed base cream and add your choice of appropriate essential oils.

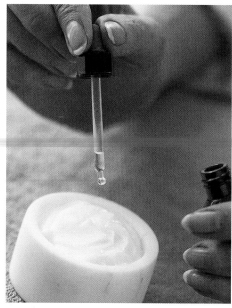

△ **1** Add a few drops of a self-prepared essential oil mix to your base cream. Use 5 drops of essential oil for every 50 ml base cream for a moisturizer.

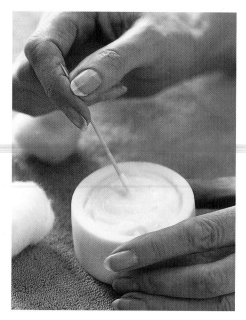

△ **2** Use a toothpick or the handle of a teaspoon to blend the oils into the cream. The prepared cream is ideal for use as a moisturizer or hand cream.

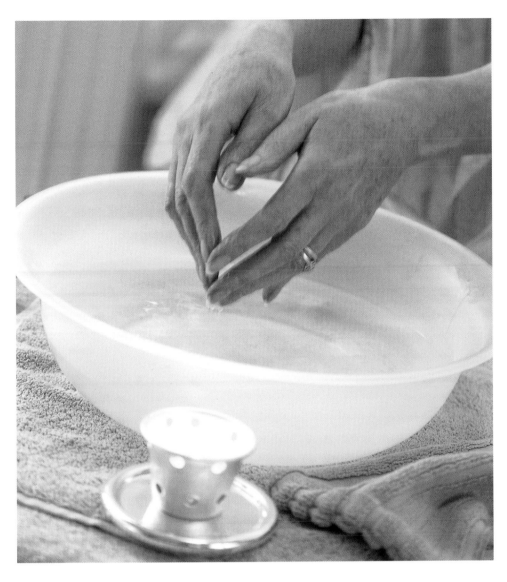

△ If it is not possible to take a full aromatherapy bath, a hand or foot bath can be as effective for arthritic hands and feet. Add a few drops of your chosen oils to warm water and soak your hands for ten to fifteen minutes.

incontinence

This upsetting condition can be helped by gentle exercise to strengthen the pelvic floor muscles. Lying on your back, tense and relax your pelvic muscles, by raising your hips 10–20 times a day, at regular intervals. Astringent essential oils can also be useful, taken internally in a tea (*see* Aromatherapy Techniques).

pressure sores

If a woman becomes bed-bound she is at risk of developing pressure sores, which are notoriously difficult to heal. To prevent these, the patient should be moved every few hours so that she is not left too long in the same position. Rub a mix of essential oils in calendula into the buttock area every day. If weeping sores develop, prepare a mineral water mix (*see* Aromatherapy Techniques) with essential oils, shake well and use to spray on to the affected area.

digestive problems

The most effective way to treat digestive disorders with essential oils is by ingestion (*see* Aromatherapy Techniques). Ideally, you should consult a qualified aromatologist. If you decide to treat yourself, it is imperative to use only genuine essential oils and to carefully follow the directions in this book.

Application of recommended essential oils can also give good results. The oils can be mixed in a carrier lotion and rubbed gently on to the abdomen in a clockwise direction, or applied on a compress and left on the abdomen overnight. Massage to the colon reflex on the feet (*see* Swiss Reflex Therapy), in a clockwise direction, can also be beneficial.

indigestion

This can occur for a number of reasons: eating too much or too quickly, eating foods which are too rich, or through emotional causes such as worry, impatience and frustration. Essential oils are excellent for indigestion. Relevant essential oils can be used in an abdominal or SRT massage every 30 minutes before a meal.

constipation

This may arise as a side-effect of medication or through emotional causes, such as fear and anxiety. Changes in environment and routine can also bring on constipation.

diarrhoea

This may be due to anxiety, fear, infections, other medication or an overdose of laxatives taken to relieve constipation.

diverticulitis

Small, harmless, thin-walled sacs can form on the colon in elderly people, through insufficient fibre in the diet. Diverticulitis is when these sacs become inflamed and painful, leading to occasional bleeding and chronic constipation. Switch to a fibre-rich diet, and use essential oils for constipation and other anti-inflammatory conditions.

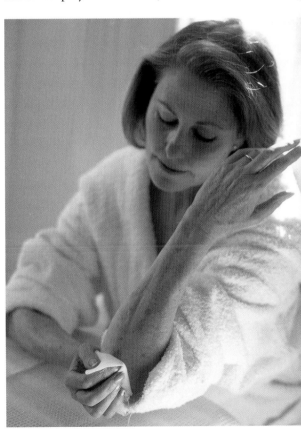

△ Lavender oil soaked into a warm compress can help to relieve the pain of arthritic joints.

Strengthening mental health

Physical health problems, minor or major, can become a source of worry and anxiety for an aging person, and can affect their overall mental and emotional health.

headaches and migraines

The reason for these, especially in the elderly, is not always apparent. It is therefore a good idea to use two or more essential oils, to make best use of their synergy. Put the relevant essential oils into your moisturizing cream and use twice daily. This helps both to relieve and prevent the problem, and will benefit the skin at the same time. If headaches persist throughout the day, try inhalation. If the headaches frequently recur, consider that it may be due to a food allergy, such as caffeine. If home treatment is unsuccessful it may be worth visiting a qualified aromatherapist.

shock

The emotional impact of shock can be particularly traumatic for an elderly person. Very often the shock is accompanied by fear, especially in the case of someone who lives on their own. Shock-induced trauma can be helped immediately by inhaling or applying essential oils with a sedative effect.

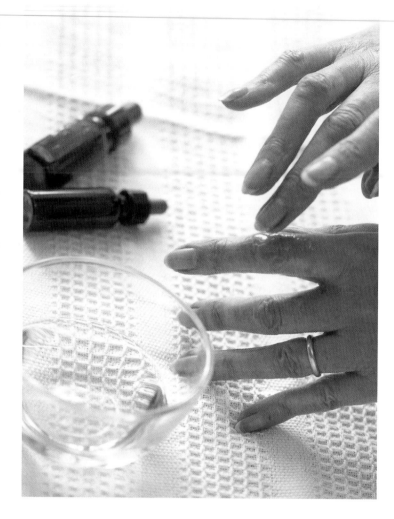

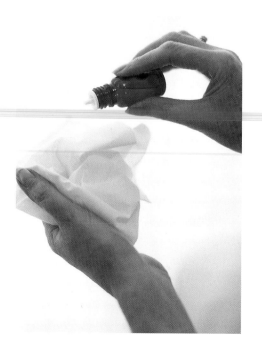

◁ Oils for fear and anger can be a useful support for cancer patients. Use juniper, lemon and geranium in a base lotion and apply the mix to the hands and body.

insomnia

Insomnia is fairly common amongst older people, and can get worse as age advances. Sometimes, there is no clear explanation for it – older people seem to need less sleep. However, the problem may be caused or exacerbated by anxiety and worry. Cramp in the leg muscles or arthritic pain during the night can also disturb the sleep pattern. The traditional essential oil used to help insomnia is lavender, although care should be taken with the dose, as too much will keep you wide awake. Lavender oil, used alone or in a synergy with two or three oils, has been used successfully by some hospitals to treat insomnia.

◁ Lavender and sweet marjoram oils can help with grief and fear. Inhale them from a tissue.

cancer

Aromatherapy cannot cure cancer but it can be used in a supportive role and can greatly improve the quality of life for many cancer patients. Fear of developing cancer can be a big worry for someone who has already lost a relative through the disease, and for cancer patients whose cancer is in remission. Use oils which are good for stress conditions (*see* Coping with Stress), and apply by inhalation, compresses and direct application in a carrier lotion.

dementia

Some people, more often in old age, suffer deterioration of their mental faculties, and are unable to think clearly or to concentrate for any length of time. The memory can become unreliable and confused, and some

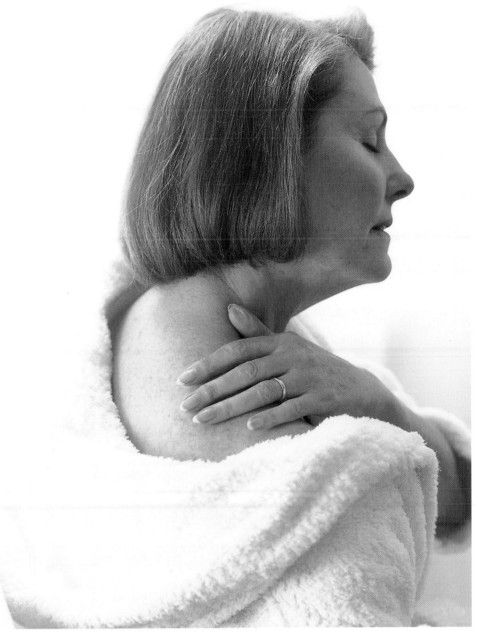

▷ Persistent headaches are debilitating and stressful. Massaging the shoulders with Roman chamomile and lavender will have a sedative and calming effect, while peppermint and rosemary will be energizing and uplifting.

speech difficulties may develop (this is particularly true after a stroke). Alzheimer's disease may develop if the nerve tissue (which cannot regenerate itself) withers and dies in the brain. Try using essential oils which stimulate the mind and improve memory. Some oils are also thought to be able to trigger past experiences, which is helpful for people with Alzheimer's.

Parkinson's disease

The cause of this debilitating, progressive disease is unknown, but a lack of the chemical substance, dopamine, which is needed for co-ordination of the brain muscles, seems to be responsible for its symptoms. Parkinson's disease is characterized by tremors, muscular rigidity and emaciation, and causes difficulty in speech and movement. Strong drugs are available to replace the dopamine; these help for a while, but they gradually lose efficiency as the body gets used to them. This necessitates a regular increase in dosage levels as the years pass, until, finally, the maximum dose loses its effect, and nothing more can be done to help the patient.

Side effects of the drugs include nausea, insomnia and constipation, all of which can be helped by aromatherapy. One study has also shown that essential oils can alleviate muscular problems, occasionally reducing the degree of slurred speech and tremors. Daily application of a lotion containing essential oils, plus daily aromatherapy baths (where possible) were used in the study. The symptoms which cause the most problems seem to be anxiety, lack of energy, muscular pains and stiffness. Others are constipation, insomnia, cramp, rigidity, tremors and slurred speech. Choose essential oils on the basis of the symptoms causing the trouble.

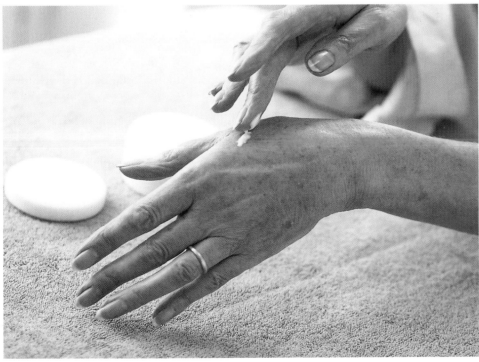

◁ For sufferers of Parkinson's disease, a hand and body lotion containing clary sage, sweet marjoram and rosemary can help the condition.

Useful essential oils

essential oil	treatment
poor circulation	
Clary sage *Salvia sclarea*	circulatory problems, haemorrhoids, varicose veins, venous aneurism, cholesterol
Lemon *Citrus limon*	poor circulation, thrombosis, varicose veins
Rosemary *Rosmarinus officinalis*	decongestant, poor circulation, hardening of the arteries
arthritis and rheumatism	
Chamomile (Roman) *Chamaemelum nobile*	anti-inflammatory, stress-relieving
Clove bud *Syzygium aromaticum*	analgesic (severe pain), anti-inflammatory, neurotonic (use sparingly - *see* The Essential Oils)
Lavender *Lavandula angustifolia*	analgesic, anti-inflammatory, stress-relieving
Marjoram (sweet) *Origanum majorana*	analgesic, stress-relieving
Niaouli *Melaleuca viridiflora*	analgesic, anti-inflammatory, neurotonic
Rosemary *Rosmarinus officinalis*	analgesic, anti-inflammatory, decongestant, neuromuscular action, neurotonic
bronchial asthma and bronchitis	
Marjoram (sweet) *Origanum majorana*	antispasmodic, anti-infectious, expels mucus, respiratory tonic
Niaouli *Melaleuca viridiflora*	anticatarrhal, anti-infectious, anti-inflammatory, expels mucus
Peppermint *Mentha* x *piperita*	anti-inflammatory, breaks down and expels mucus
Pine *Pinus sylvestris*	analgesic, anti-infectious, anti-inflammatory, decongestant, breaks down and expels mucus
Rosemary *Rosmarinus officinalis*	breaks down mucus, anti-inflammatory, decongestant, expels mucus
headaches	
Chamomile (Roman) *Chamaemelum nobile*	antispasmodic, calming, sedative
Lavender *Lavandula angustifolia*	analgesic, calming, sedative
Marjoram (sweet) *Origanum majorana*	analgesic, antispasmodic, calming
Melissa *Melissa officinalis*	calming, sedative
Peppermint *Mentha* x *piperita*	analgesic, antispasmodic
Rosemary *Rosmarinus officinalis*	analgesic, antispasmodic, decongestant

essential oil	treatment
influenza	
Eucalyptus *Eucalyptus smithii*	anti-infectious, antiviral, prophylactic
Cypress *Cupressus sempervirens*	anti-infectious
Lemon *Citrus limon*	anti-infectious, antiviral
Pine *Pinus sylvestris*	anti-infectious
insomnia	
Basil *Ocimum basilicum* var. *album*	nervous system regulator (nervous insomnia)
Chamomile (Roman) *Chamaemelum nobile*	calming
Lavender *Lavandula angustifolia*	calming, sedative
Lemon *Citrus limon*	calming
Marjoram (sweet) *Origanum majorana*	calming
Melissa *Melissa officinalis*	calming, sedative
shock	
Bergamot *Citrus bergamia*	balancing, calming, sedative, tonic to central nervous system
Chamomile (Roman) *Chamaemelum nobile*	calming, sedative
Lavender *Lavandula angustifolia*	balancing, calming, sedative, tonic
Melissa *Melissa officinalis*	calming, sedative
incontinence	
Cypress *Cupressus sempervirens*	astringent
Lemon *Citrus limon*	astringent
pressure sores	
Chamomile (German) *Matricaria recutica*	cicatrizant (infected wounds, ulcers)
Chamomile (Roman) *Chamaemelum nobile*	vulnerary (boils, burns wounds).
Frankincense *Boswellia carteri*	cicatrizant (scars, ulcers, wounds)
Geranium *Pelargonium graveolens*	cicatrizant (burns, cuts, ulcers, wounds)
Lavender *Lavandula angustifolia*	cicatrizant (burns, scars, varicose veins, wounds)
constipation and diverticulitis	
Ginger *Zingiber officinale*	analgesic, digestive stimulant, general tonic
Mandarin *Citrus reticulata*	antispasmodic, calming, digestive.
Orange (bitter) *Citrus aurantium* var. *amara*	calming, digestive

essential oil	treatment
Rosemary *Rosmarinus officinalis*	analgesic, anti-inflammatory, digestive (constipation, sluggish or painful digestion)

diarrhoea

essential oil	treatment
Geranium *Pelargonium graveolens*	anti-inflammatory (colitis), anti-spasmodic (colic, gastroenteritis), astringent
Lemon *Citrus limon*	antispasmodic, astringent, stomachic (gastritis, stomach ulcers).
Marjoram (sweet) *Origanum majorana*	analgesic, anti-infectious, anti-spasmodic (colic), stomachic (enteritis)
Niaouli *Melaleuca viridiflora*	anti-infectious, anti-inflammatory, antiviral (viral enteritis), digestive (gastritis)
Peppermint *Mentha* x *piperita*	anti-infectious, anti-inflammatory (colitis, enteritis, gastritis), antispasmodic (gastric spasm), digestive

indigestion (dyspepsia)

essential oil	treatment
Basil *Ocimum basilicum* var. *album*	analgesic, carminative (flatulence, sluggish digestion)
Lemon *Citrus limon*	digestive (nausea, painful digestion, flatulence, appetite loss)
Marjoram (sweet) *Origanum majorana*	analgesic, calming, digestive – (flatulence, indigestion)
Orange (bitter) *Citrus aurantium* var. *amara*	calming, digestive
Peppermint *Mentha* x *piperita*	analgesic, carminative (flatulence), digestive (nausea, painful digestion)
Rosemary *Rosmarinus officinalis*	analgesic (painful digestion), carminative (flatulence)

dementia and Alzheimer's disease

essential oil	treatment
Basil *Ocimum basilicum* var. *album*	neurotonic (mental strain)
Clove bud *Syzygium aromaticum*	mental stimulant (memory loss, mental fatigue), neurotonic
Marjoram (sweet) *Origanum majorana*	neurotonic (mental instability)
Peppermint *Mentha* x *piperita*	mental stimulant (concentration), neurotonic
Rosemary *Rosmarinus officinalis*	neurotonic (loss of memory, concentration)

Parkinson's disease

essential oil	treatment
Clary sage *Salvia sclarea*	antispasmodic, calming, regenerative (cellular aging), neurotonic
Lavender *Lavandula angustifolia*	analgesic, antispasmodic, calming, sedative (anxiety, headaches, insomnia), neurotonic
Marjoram (sweet) *Origanum majorana*	analgesic, antispasmodic, digestive tonic, calming (anxiety, insomnia),
Rosemary *Rosmarinus officinalis*	analgesic, antispasmodic, digestive (constipation, sluggish digestion), neurotonic

...'Tis the hour

That scatters spells on herb and flower

And garlands might be gathered now

That turn'd around the sleeper's brow.

From Light of the Haram, Thomas Moore, 1779–1852.

References

the teenage years

Ball, J. (1990) *Understanding Disease*, Daniel, Saffron Walden.

Brown, F. (1986) *Skin Care*, Springhouse, P.A.

Cohen, E. L., Pegum, J. S. (1970) *Dermatology*, Baillére, Tindall and Cassel.

Hartvig & Rowley (1996) *You Are What You Eat*, Paitkus.

Price, L. (1985) *Scalp Problems* (notes), Shirley Price International College of Aromatherapy.

Stanway, P. (1989) *Diet For Common Ailments*, Gaia Books.

Trusty, L. S. (1969) *The Art and Science of Barbering*, Self-published.

Wingate P., Wingate R. (1988) *The Penguin Medical Encyclopedia*, Penguin.

beauty and well-being

Ball, J. (1987) *Understanding Disease*, Blackdown.

Collin, P. H. (1994) *Directory Of Medicine*, Peter Collin Publishing.

Domar, A. D., Drehar, H. (1997) *Healing Mind, Healthy Woman*, Thorsons.

Fischer-Rizzi, S. (1990) *Complete Aromatherapy Handbook*, Sterling.

Gatti, G., Cayola, R. (1923) *Therapeutic Action of Essential Oils*, Revista Italiana delle Essenze e Profumi.

Hall-Smith, P., Cairns, R. J., Beare, R. L. B. (1973) *Dermatology*, Crosby, Lockwood, Staples.

Jäger, W., Buchbauer, G., Jirovetz, L., Fritzer, M. (1992) *Percutaneous Absorption Of Lavender Oil From A Massage Oil*, Journal of the Society of Cosmetic Chemists.

Price, S. (2000) *Aromatherapy and The Emotions*, Thorsons.

Price, S. (1999) *Practical Aromatherapy* (4th edition), Thorsons.

Ratcliffe, J. D. (1992) *I Am Joe's Body*, Berkley.

Wood, C. (1990) *Say Yes To Life*, Dent.

the reproductive years

Balacs, T. (1992) *Safety In Pregnancy*, International Journal of Aromatherapy.

Domar, A., Drehar, H. (1997) *Healing Mind, Healthy Woman*, Thorsons.

Franchomme, P., Pénoël, D. (1990) *L'aromathérapie Exactement*, Jollois.

Freeman, H. (1994) *Essential Oils and Problems Related To The Menstrual Cycle*, The Aromatherapist (Vol. 3, 2).

Guenier, J. (1992) *Essential Obstetrics*, International Journal Of Aromatherapy.

Myles, M. (1993) *Textbook For Midwives* (12th edition), Churchill Livingstone.

Price, S. (1999) *Practical Aromatherapy* (5th edition), Thorsons.

Valnet, J. (1980) *The Practice Of Aromatherapy*, Daniel, Saffron Walden.

Wingate, P., Wingate, R. (1988) *The Penguin Medical Encyclopedia*, Penguin Books.

Worwood, V. (1990) *The Fragrant Pharmacy*, MacMillan.

the menopause

Ball, J. (1987) *Understanding Disease*, Blackdown.

Domar, A., Drehar, H. (1997) *Healing Mind, Healthy Woman*, Thorsons.

Slade, J. (1994) *The Menopause*, The Aromatherapist (Vol. 1).

Wyatt, T. (1999) *The Menopause* (unpublished paper), Shirley Price International College of Aromatherapy.

the sunset years

Buckle, J. (1997) *Clinical Aromatherapy In Nursing*, Arnold.

Price, S., Price, L. (1999) *Aromatherapy For Health Professionals* (2nd edition), Churchill Livingstone.

Price, S. (1999) *Practical Aromatherapy* (4th edition), Thorsons.

Wingate, P., Wingate, R. (1988) *Penguin Medical Encyclopedia*, Penguin.

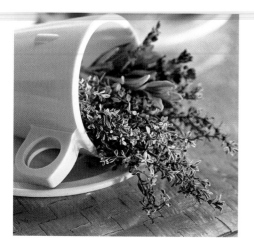

Glossary

analgesic reduces sensitivity to pain.

anaphrodisiac diminishes sexual drive.

antiallergic reduces sensitivity to various substances.

antibacterial agent which kills bacteria.

anticoagulant agent which stops blood from clotting.

antidiabetic prevents the development of diabetes.

antifungal prevents the development of fungus.

anti-inflammatory reduces inflammation.

antilactogenic prevents or slows down the secretion of milk in nursing mothers.

antimigraine reduces or prevents migraines.

antiparasitic prevents the development of parasites.

antipruritic relieves itching.

antipyretic counteracts inflammation or fever.

antisclerotic antiageing; prevents hardening of tissues.

antiseptic prevents the development of bacteria.

antispasmodic prevents muscle spasm, convulsion.

antitussive relieves or prevents coughing.

antiviral prevents the development of viruses.

aperitif stimulates the appetite.

aphrodisiac arouses sexual desire.

aromatology the study of essential oils for health, including intensive and internal use.

astringent causes contraction of living tissue.

balsamic fragrant substance that softens phlegm.

capillary dilator dilates the capillaries, aids circulation.

cardiotonic has a tonic effect on the heart.

carminative relieves flatulence (wind).

chemotype visually identical plants with significantly different chemical components and properties, e.g. *Thyme vulgaris* phenol and alcohol chemotypes.

choleretic stimulates bile production in the liver.

cicatrizant healing; promotes scar tissue.

decongestant relieves congestion in the skin, digestive, circulatory and respiratory systems.

depurative purifying or cleansing.

diaphoretic see sudorific.

digestive stimulant stimulates a sluggish digestion.

diuretic promotes the secretion of urine.

emmenagogic induces or regularizes menstruation.

essential oil volatile plant oil obtained only by distillation (exception: oil obtained by expression of the peel of citrus fruits).

febrifuge reduces temperature; antipyretic.

fixed oil non-volatile vegetable oil.

hypertensor increases blood pressure in hypotensive person.

hypotensor reduces blood pressure in hypertensive person.

lactogen promotes the secretion of milk.

laxative loosens the bowel contents.

lipolytic breaks down fat.

litholytic breaks down sand or small kidney or urinary stones.

maceration the extraction of components from plants by steeping in fixed oil.

mucolytic breaks down mucus and catarrh.

neurotonic stimulates and tones the nervous system.

oestrogenic simulates the action of the female hormone, oestrogen.

phlebotonic improves or stimulates lymph circulation; lymph tonic.

prophylactic prevents disease.

rubefacient increases local blood circulation causing redness of the skin.

stomachic stimulates secretory activity in the stomach.

styptic arrests haemorrhage by means of astringent quality; haemostatic.

sudorific induces or increases perspiration.

synergy the working together that occurs when two or more substances used together give a more effective result than the same substances used alone.

uterotonic improves the tone of the uterus (womb).

vasodilator causes blood vessels to increase in lumen (the hollow inside of the blood vessel).

vulnerary promotes the healing of wounds.

Useful addresses

UNITED KINGDOM
Aromatherapy associations
Aromatherapy Organizations Council
(AOC)
P. O. Box 19834
London SE25 6WF
Tel: 020 8251 7912

International Society of Professional
Aromatherapists (ISPA)
ISPA House
82 Ashby Road
Hinckley
Leics LE10 1SN
Tel: 01455 647 987

International Federation of
Aromatherapists (IFA)
Stamford House
2–4 Chiswick High Street
London W4 1TH
Tel: 020 8742 2605

Aromatherapy products
Shirley Price Aromatherapy Limited
Essentia House
Upper Bond Street
Hinckley
Leics LE10 1RS
Tel: 01455 615 466

Herbal Garden
93 Rose Street
Edinburgh EH2 3DT
Tel: 0131 220 0251

Specialized short courses in aromatherapy
Penny Price
Sketchley Manor
Burbage
Leics LE10 2LQ
Fax: 01455 617 972

Aromatic medicine and aromatology
Dr Robert Stephen
4 Woodland Road
Hinckley
Leics LE10 1JG
Telefax: 01455 611 829

UNITED STATES
Aromatherapy associations
Nordbloom Swedish Healthcare Center
178 Mill Creek Road
Livingstone
Montana 59047
Tel: 406 333 4216

The Australasian College of
Herbal Studies
P. O. Box 57
Lake Oswego
Oregon 97034
Tel: 503 635 6652

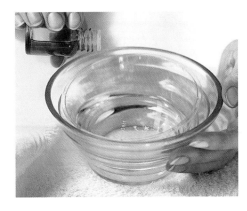

NORTHERN IRELAND
Aromatherapy products
Angela Hills
32 Russell Park
Belfast BT5 7QW

REPUBLIC OF IRELAND
Aromatherapy products
Chritine Courtney
Oban Aromatherapy
53 Beech Grove
Lucan
County Dublin

NORWAY
Aromatherapy products
Margareth Thomte
Nedreslottsgate 25
0157 Oslo
Tel: 22 170017

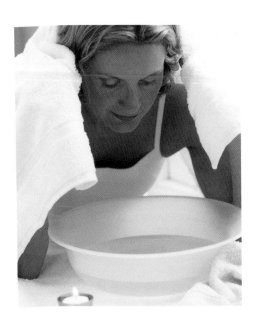

Acknowledgements

My first thanks must go to God, who has been with me every step of the way. I would also like to thank my husband, Len, and my son-in-law, Robert, for their help and advice, and my daughter, Penny, who acted as consultant at the photography sessions. Thanks, too, to Sarah Ainley, my link with Anness Publishing, who has been very patient with me!

The publishers and photographer would like to thank the following models for their contribution: Anneke Swenska, Alex Cameron, Debbie Grieve, Kerry Cleave, Janice Harris, Joanna Dove, Joy Harris, Nancy Markwick and Sarah Raine.

Index

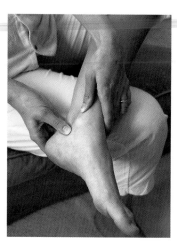

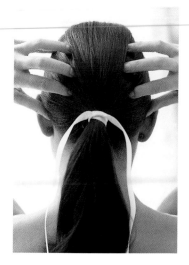